T0076163

CARDIOLOGY RESEARCH AND CLINICAL DEVELOPMENTS

CHEST PAIN: CAUSES, DIAGNOSIS, AND TREATMENT

CARDIOLOGY RESEARCH AND CLINICAL DEVELOPMENTS

Additional books in this series can be found on Nova's website under the Series tab.

Additional E-books in this series can be found on Nova's website under the E-books tab.

CARDIOLOGY RESEARCH AND CLINICAL DEVELOPMENTS

CHEST PAIN: CAUSES, DIAGNOSIS, AND TREATMENT

SOPHIE M. WEBER
EDITOR

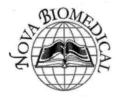

Nova Science Publishers, Inc.
New York

Library of Congress Cataloging-in-Publication Data

Chest pain : causes, diagnosis, and treatment / editor, Sophie M. Weber.
 p. ; cm.
Includes bibliographical references and index.
ISBN 978-1-61728-112-9 (hardcover)
1. Chest pain. I. Weber, Sophie M.
[DNLM: 1. Angina Pectoris. 2. Chest Pain. WG 298 C5245 2010]
RC941.C572 2010
616.1'22--dc22
                                    2010016739

Published by Nova Science Publishers, Inc. ✦ *New York*

Contents

Preface

Chest pain may be a symptom of a number of serious conditions and is generally considered a medical emergency. Even though it may be determined that the pain is non-cardiac in origin, this is often a diagnosis of exclusion made after ruling out more serious causes of the pain. This new book gathers and presents topical data on the causes, diagnosis and treatment of chest pain including integrated studies of western and traditional Chinese medicine on Cardiac Syndrome X with chest pain, angina and chest pain, a look at the available prediction instruments that can be used for the classification of acute coronary syndrome (ACS), and ambient nitrogen dioxide and female emergency room visits for chest pain.

Chapter 1- Cardiac Syndrome X (CSX) is a kind of clinical syndrome with typical symptoms of angina pectoris, positive result of electrocardiogram (ECG) and/or treadmill exercise test, negative result of coronary angiography (CAG), and no coronary artery spasm, which is also known as "Microvascular Angina" . In recent years, clinical reports on CSX have been increasing, but the pathogenesis of CSX is still not quite clear. By now, although a variety of clinical drugs and means have been utilized in the treatment for CSX, most of which could just relieve symptoms and not be good to improve the quality of life greatly or even cure the disease completely. Therefore, there are still necessary for chasing more effective treatment programs.

The traditional Chinese medicine (TCM) may be a new effective approach for the prevention and treatment of CSX. TCM therapies showed a certain efficacy advantage in improving clinical symptoms and quality of life for the CSX patients. From the perspective of our TCM studies, chest pain is the main manifestations of CSX, and Qi stagnation, phlegm retention and blood stasis are the mostly TCM typical syndrome patterns for CSX. "Qi-regulating, chest-relaxing and blood-activating" is the main TCM treatment method. The clinical trial indicated that Qi-regulating, chest-relaxing and blood-activating therapy could reduce the frequency and degree of the occurrence of angina, as well as improve patients' TCM syndromes and exercise tolerance. Meanwhile, the treatment method could inhibit inflammatory response of vascular wall and protect the function of vascular endothelial cell.

Chapter 2- Despite decades of health outcomes research, a fail-safe way to rule out acute coronary syndrome (ACS) at the time of a patient's initial presentation remains elusive. Although there may be variability in the rates at which ACS is missed at individual hospitals, the "missed ACS rate" is generally inversely proportional to the rule-in rate. Predicting the patients who will ultimately be diagnosed with ACS is particularly problematic for that subset of patients with acute chest pain but with normal initial cardiac biomarkers and a non-diagnostic electrocardiogram.

This chapter will summarize the available prediction instruments that can be used for likelihood classification of ACS, including the most contemporary risk scores. How these tools address the need for intensive care and predict short-term prognosis will be explored. Data comparing these scores will also be reviewed. Lastly, a discussion of the pros, cons, and applications of several validated models to classify the presence or absence of ACS in undifferentiated ED populations will be presented.

Chapter 3- Body surface potential mapping was first described by Flowers and Horan, as a method to obtain more extensive and precise information than that provided by the standard 12-lead electrocardiogram (ECG) [1]. Although the dipole model for cardiac electrical activity accounts for ~80% of the hearts electrical activity, in reality this electrical field is much more complex and contains multiple areas of positive and negative potential. Thus, body surface mapping allows a more comprehensive representation of cardiac myocyte depolarisation and repolarisation.

Body surface mapping permits correlation of body surface and epimyocardial events: Monro and colleagues successfully demonstrated a correlation between epicardial recordings from temporary pacing wires post-cardiac surgery and surface recordings using a 37-lead ECG [2]. Furthermore, body surface mapping allows detection of events not detectable by the conventional 12-lead ECG. In 1993, Kornreich *et al* compared body surface maps (BSM) in 131 patients with acute myocardial infarction (76 anterior, 32 inferior, 23 posterior) from 159 normal controls using a 120-lead BSM and discriminant function technique (Table 1).

Chapter 4- Chest pain has a wide differential diagnosis. It is well recognized as a common presentation of acute coronary ischemia. Despite availability of multiple diagnostic modalities for evaluation of chest pain, the rate of missed myocardial infarction ranges from 2%-10% [1, 2] A patient with known coronary atherosclerotic disease remains at high risk for recurrent coronary events. Nonetheless, similar to any other patient presenting with chest pain, a systematic diagnostic approach is needed. Listening to the patient's description of symptoms is important.

The earliest description of effort angina by William Heberden over 200 years ago still holds true [3]. He described it as *"a disorder of the breast marked with strong and peculiar symptoms. The seat of it, and sense of strangling, and anxiety with which it is attended, may make it not improperly called angina pectoris. Those who are afflicted with it are seized while they are walking and more particularly when they walk soon after eating with painful and most disagreeable sensations in the breast which seems as if it would take their life away if it were to increase or continue. The moment they stand still all this uneasiness vanishes".*

Chapter 5- Angina is one of the commonest causes of chest pain. It is a common initial manifestation of coronary heart disease, a significant burden in primary care and has considerable economic implications globally. Angina is usually diagnosed from a clinical constellation of symptoms from the patient's history. Descriptions of symptoms, articulated by patients to their doctors, remain a cornerstone of diagnosis in clinical medicine. Whilst the diagnosis of angina is straight forward in many cases, it can be difficult in certain circumstances such as older people and people presenting with atypical symptoms. There have been recent developments in European guidelines for the diagnosis of angina. In this chapter we will describe the definition, causes of angina and its differential diagnosis. We will also discuss its management from primary and secondary prevention and treatment perspectives.

Chapter 6- *Objectives*: Ambient exposure to nitrogen dioxide (NO_2) has been previously associated with the occurrence of chest pain. The objective of the current study was to examine the correlation between ambient nitrogen dioxide concentrations and emergency department (ED) visits for chest pain in Toronto, Canada. *Design and Methods*: This was a case-crossover study of ED visits for chest pain in female patients that were recorded at one hospital. In the constructed conditional logistic regression models, temperature and relative humidity were adjusted in the form of natural splines with 3 degrees of freedom. The calculations were completed for a sequence of 47 overlapping age groups: [20, 39], [21, 40], and so on, up to [66, 85]. The results, expressed as odds ratios (ORs) and their respective 95% confidence intervals (95% CI), were reported for an increase in the interquartile range (IQR = 75th − 25th percentiles; IQR = 9.9 ppb). *Results:* The results were summarized in two figures. One figure shows the OR values and their respective 95% CIs; another represents median values and two quartiles (1 and 3) for controls and cases, both for 47 age groups. Positive and statistically significant associations were observed for patients in the age interval [39, 72] years; the OR = 1.10 (95% CI: 1.00, 1.22). *Conclusions:* Our findings provide additional support for an association between NO_2 exposure and the number of ED visits for chest pain in female patients.

In: Chest Pain Causes, Diagnosis and Treatment   ISBN 978-1-61728-112-9
Editor: Sophie M. Weber, pp. 1-34   © 2010 Nova Science Publishers, Inc.

Chapter 1

Integrated Studies of Western and Traditional Chinese Medicine on Cardiac Syndrome X, One Kind of Diseases with Chest Pain

*Jingyuan Mao[*1], Yingfei Bi[†2], Xianliang Wang[‡1], Henghe Wang[•1], Yongbin Ge[»1], and Zhenpeng Zhang[^3]*

[1].Cardiovascular Department of The First Teaching Hospital of Tianjin University of Traditional Chinese Medicine Tianjin, China

[2.]Tianjin University of Traditional Chinese Medicine, Tianjin, China

[3]Cardiovascular Department of Guang An Men Hospital of Chinese Scientific Academy of Traditional Chinese Medicine, Beijing, China

Abstract

Cardiac Syndrome X (CSX) is a kind of clinical syndrome with typical symptoms of angina pectoris, positive result of electrocardiogram (ECG) and/or treadmill exercise test, negative result of coronary angiography (CAG), and no coronary artery spasm, which is also known

[*] Corresponding author: Mao Jingyuan, Telephone: 86-022-27432325, Email addresses: jymao@126.com.
[†] #312 Anshan Western Road, Nankai District, Tianjin, China. Email addresses: yingfei1981@163.com.
[‡] xlwang1981@126.com.
[•] henghewang@126.com.
[»] geyongbin66@yahoo.com.cn.
[^] #5 Beixiange, Xuanwu District, Beijing, China. Email addresses: zzpshou@163.com.

as "Microvascular Angina" . In recent years, clinical reports on CSX have been increasing, but the pathogenesis of CSX is still not quite clear. By now, although a variety of clinical drugs and means have been utilized in the treatment for CSX, most of which could just relieve symptoms and not be good to improve the quality of life greatly or even cure the disease completely. Therefore, there are still necessary for chasing more effective treatment programs.

The traditional Chinese medicine (TCM) may be a new effective approach for the prevention and treatment of CSX. TCM therapies showed a certain efficacy advantage in improving clinical symptoms and quality of life for the CSX patients. From the perspective of our TCM studies, chest pain is the main manifestations of CSX, and Qi stagnation, phlegm retention and blood stasis are the mostly TCM typical syndrome patterns for CSX. "Qi-regulating, chest-relaxing and blood-activating" is the main TCM treatment method. The clinical trial indicated that Qi-regulating, chest-relaxing and blood-activating therapy could reduce the frequency and degree of the occurrence of angina, as well as improve patients' TCM syndromes and exercise tolerance. Meanwhile, the treatment method could inhibit inflammatory response of vascular wall and protect the function of vascular endothelial cell.

Introduction

Cardiac Syndrome X (CSX) is a kind of clinical syndrome with typical symptoms of angina, positive result of electrocardiogram (ECG) and/or treadmill exercise test, negative result of coronary angiography (CAG), and no coronary artery spasm, which is also known as "Microvascular Angina".

In 1967, American scholars Likoff W and his colleagues reported such cases for the first time, and referred to as "angina pectoris with normal coronary arteries" [1]. Kemp HG named it as "X syndrome" in 1973 [2]. Cannon RO proposed that the chest pain in CSX patients was induced by myocardial ischemia resulted from the dysfunction of small coronary blood vessels (<500um), and suggested it was known as microvascular angina [3]. With typical angina and positive result of treadmill exercise test, 10% ~ 30% patients were found no significant vascular stenosis by cardiac catheterization [4]. These patients were often diagnosed as cardiac syndrome X.

Section 1 Pathogenesis of CSX

The pathogenesis of CSX is not quite clear at present. It may be induced by a variety of factors, including the reduction of the coronary flow reserve, endothelial dysfunction, abnormal pain perception, inflammation, estrogen deficiency, emotional factors, atherosclerosis, and so on. What we have summarized are as follows.

1. Reduction of the Coronary Flow Reserve

Coronary flow reserve (CFR) is the ratio between the maximum and the basis of coronary blood flow. Normal CFR level is 2.5~5 times higher than the basis level. The decline of CFR is often prompted that the myocardial blood supply can not increase correspondingly when activity, which may be one of the reasons for the angina of CSX patients.

Many tests were designed to induce angina pectoris, through intravenous injection of vasodilator drugs (dipyridamole, nitroglycerin, papaverine, adenosine, etc) or cardiac stress test (such as exercise testing, dobutamine test, etc). The results showed that the patients with CSX commonly had myocardial blood perfusion abnormalities and reduction, by using Doppler ultrasound, emission computerized tomography (ECT), cardiac magnetic resonance (CMR) or position emission tomography (PET), etc. [5-15]

2. Endothelial Dysfunction

Current studies suggest coronary endothelial cell dysfunction is the leading cause of CSX. Microvascular abnormalities, caused by endothelial dysfunction, appear to be responsible for myocardial ischemia in patients with CSX. Endothelial dysfunction is likely to be multifactorial in CSX patients and it is conceivable that risk factors such as hypertension, hypercholesterolemia, obesity, diabetes mellitus, metabolic syndrome, smoking, inflammation, estrogen deficiency and insulin resistance could contribute to its development.

Normally, endothelial cells regulate blood flow through coronary microcirculation by releasing dilating and constricting factors. Dilating factors include nitric oxide (NO) and prostacyclin, and constricting factors include endothelin-1(ET-1) and angiotensin II (AT II). These factors directly affect muscles in the cardiac vessels by increasing or decreasing lumen size and the amount of blood in coronary microcirculation. In coronary endothelial cell dysfunction, there may be excessive constricting factors or not enough dilating factors. The vasoconstrictive effect can not be antagonistic by NO, which results in endothelium-dependent vasodilation (EDV) obstacled, myocardial blood flow reduced, microvascular ischemia and chest pain occured finally. Furthermore, recent insights suggested that the injured endothelial monolayer was regenerated by circulating bone marrow-derived endothelial progenitor cells (EPCs). These findings of studies on EPCs may explain the underlying mechanisms which contribute to the endothelial dysfunction and microvascular abnormalities observed in patients with CSX. [16-28]

3. Neural Factors and Abnormal Pain Perception

The normal function of the cardiovascular system is regulated by the sympathetic and parasympathetic system, and the disorders of central nervous system can induce cardiovascular dysfunction. The studies found, CSX patients were often accompanied by increased sensitivity to pain stimulation, and the nervous system may play an important role to lead to the abnormal pain perception. The imbalance of nerve regulating function may be one of the causes to the persistent chest pain in CSX patients. [29-32]

4. Inflammatory Response

Systemic inflammation is a potential physiologic cause of CSX. The relationship between inflammatory response and CSX has been generally supported by many studies on the mechanism of inflammatory substances, such as high sensitivity C reactive protein(hs-CRP), intercellular adhesion molecule-1(ICAM-1), vascular cell adhesion molecule-1(VCAM-1), interleukin-1(IL-1), tumor necrosis factor-α(TNF-α), interferon-γ(IFN-γ), helicobacter pylori(H.pylori), and so on. The mechanisms of these inflammatory substances on CSX were likely to complicate endothelial cell function, hinder the release of dilating factors, and lead to EDV obstacle, thereby limiting blood flow to the heart and leading to chest pain. [33-41]

5. Estrogen Deficiency

In 2004, the American Heart Association (AHA) and the U.S. National Heart, Lung and Blood Institute(NHLBI) reported 60%-70% CSX patients were women, of which 60% were postmenopausal women. Estrogen deficiency may be another potential cause of CSX. Endothelial cell dysfunction, caused by estrogen deficiency, may disrupt the balance of coronary dilating and constricting factors, as well as amplify pain perception in patients with CSX. For these CSX patients, short-term estrogen given could increase coronary artery blood flow and improve EDV obstacle. [42-46]

6. Psychological Factors

The vast majority of CSX patients, especially postmenopausal women, have psychological problems. The studies found that these patients with emotional abnormalities often accompanied with more depression, anxiety and somatic concerns than positive angiographic patients. They had high scores on psychological inventories that measure anxiety and depression, and were very prone to somatization. Psychological factors may also participate in the pathogenesis of CSX and could be a pathophysiological mechanism for the cardiac chest pain of CSX patients. [47-51]

7. Atherosclerosis

The cause of myocardial ischemia and chest pain in patients with CSX has been explained by mechanisms including endothelial dysfunction. CSX patients have higher levels of asymmetric dimethylarginine (ADMA) and increased mean common carotid intima-media thickness (C-IMT), reflecting the presence of subclinical atherosclerosis. Besides endothelial dysfunction, presence of atherosclerosis may also contribute to the etiopathogenesis of the CSX phenomenon. The atherosclerotic plaques disrupt endothelial cell function, narrow arteries, and restrict blood flow. Even though diffuse plaques of microcirculation are not seen by coronary angiography, they can now be identified by intravascular coronary ultrasound. [52]

8. High Homocysteine Level

There are studies to investigate the plasma homocysteine level and the relationship between plasma homocysteine level and duke treadmill score (DTS) in CSX patients. Plasma homocysteine level, known to cause endothelial dysfunction and microvascular ischemia, is higher in CSX patients. Also, this increase in homocysteine level inversely correlates with the DTS, which represents the magnitude of ischemia. [53-54]

In addition, the incidence of CSX may also be relevant with insulin resistance [55-56], platelet size [57], hematological factors [58], lymphocyte DNA damage [59], paraoxonase, aryl esterase activity and oxidative stress [60] and other factors.

In conclusion, CSX is one disease resulted from a variety of pathogenic factors. The pathogenesis of CSX is complicated, and clarifying its pathogenesis can help to improve diagnosis and treatment level of the disease. The studies on the pathogenesis of CSX still need to be further explored.

Section 2 Diagnosis for CSX

Pupita proposed the diagnostic standards of CSX as follows: symptoms of angina pectoris, positive exercise test, and transient ST-segment depression in Holter tests [61]. Some other scholars believed that angina pectoris without ST-T changes also belong to the diagnosis [62]. Although diagnostic criteria are not universally accepted, CSX is most often diagnosed by[63-64]:

a) The presence of chest pain;
b) ST segment changes on ECG, and/or positive exercise test;
c) Normal coronary arteries as evidenced by angiography.

As "other and unspecified angina pectoris", CSX is most appropriately placed under the International Classification of Diseases (ICD). Patients, who have coronary artery spasm, left ventricular hypertrophy, diabetes mellitus, uncontrolled systemic hypertension, variant angina, cardiomyopathies, or heart valve disease, are excluded from the diagnosis of CSX, as these can provide an identifiable cause for chest pain [65].

Chest pain is the main manifestation of CSX, and may radiate to the neck, jaw, left shoulder, arms, or back. Chest pain in CSX is described as aching, squeezing, burning, heaviness, or pressure, and can range from mild to severe, occur at rest or with exertion, and last for several hours [66]. Additional subtle symptoms can include shortness of breath, lightheadedness, nausea, or cold sweats. If the requirement of ST segment changes was removed, and diagnosis based on clinical presentation, those with mild symptoms could benefit from treatment. Unfortunately, when angiography reveals clear arteries, many patients are falsely reassured of a healthy heart and are therefore offered no options for treatment [67].

Section 3 Treatment of Western Medicine for CSX

Although CSX does not result in an increased risk of cardiovascular mortality, the symptoms are often troublesome and unresponsive to conventional antianginal therapy. Not only can CSX affect the patient's quality of life, resulting in continuing episodes of chest pain and frequent hospital readmissions, but also cause a waste of medical resources and increase the patient's incidence rates of cardiovascular and cerebrovascular events. As a result, the treatment for CSX is very important and meaningful.

Understanding the underlying mechanism of disease is of vital importance for patients' management. However, the pathogenesis of CSX is not very clear at present. Though there are many potential causative factors for CSX, it is difficult to know which treatment to implement. Management of this syndrome represents a major challenge to the treating physician. Currently, the treatment of western medicine for CSX is mainly focusing on pain relief and symptomatic improvement.

Medications are the most common treatment and can reduce the severity and duration of chest pain. Conventional therapies with antianginal agents, such as nitrates, calcium channel blockers, β-blockers, have been tried with variable success. More effective therapies should be studied.. With the presence of supporting evidence for the important role of endothelial dysfunction in CSX pathogenesis, the treatments that target improving endothelial function, such as statins, angiotensin-converting enzyme inhibitors, and estrogen replacement, are increasingly used in clinical practice. Other treatment options include neurostimulation, spinal cord stimulation, psychological interventions and enhanced external counterpulsation. In addition, lifestyle modification is also important for the treatment of CSX, with avoiding tobacco, limiting alcohol drinks, controlling weight, and so on.

1. Medications

(1) Nitrates

Nitrates are vascular vasodilating, anti-ischemic and antianginal medications. They have been the
traditional mainstay of CSX therapy. However, there are many opposite voices about nitrates for CSX. Lanza GA reported sublingual nitrates could not improve the exercise tolerance in patients with syndrome X and suggested that a deficiency in coronary prearteriolar nitric oxide production was unlikely to play a key role in the pathophysiology of the syndrome [68]. Radice M also found that sublingual nitroglycerin could not improve the exercise tolerance and electrocardiogram ST-segment depression significantly [69]. It was reported that nitrates were effective only for 40% ~ 50% CSX patients and its placebo effect could not be ruled out [70].

(2) β-Blockers

β-blockers are antihypertensive medications, which can reduce heart rate and cardiac output, lower peripheral vascular resistance, slow renin release, and decrease venous return. β-blockers is also one of the most effective anti-ischemic medications. Lanza GA compared the efficacy of aβ-blockers (atenolol), a calcium antagonist (amlodipine), and a nitrate (isosorbide-5-mononitrate) on CXS patients and only atenolol was found to significantly improve chest pain episodes [71]. Sen N had one piece of opinion that nebivolol treatment was associated with better improvements in both circulating endothelial function and exercise stress test parameters than metoprolol [72]. Erdamar H also found oxidative stress and antioxidant status were ameliorated in CSX patients who had taken nebivolol in contrast to metoprolol [73]. Nebivolol treatment may be a novel treatment strategy in cases with CSX in the future.

(3) Calcium Channel Blockers

Calcium channel blockers, also known as calcium antagonists, commonly work by lowering heart rate, reducing myocardial contractility, relaxing arteriolar smooth muscle, and decrease peripheral vascular resistance. Long-term studies showed calcium channel blockers were effective against CSX pain in 31% of cases when used as monotherapy [63]. On the other hand, there are also controversies that calcium channel blockers can not improve the coronary flow reserve and reduce chest pain in CSX patients, so the utilization of calcium antagonists in clinic is not supported regularly [74].

Nitrates, β-blockers and calcium channel blockers, all belonged to anti-ischemic medications, are commonly used in the treatment of CSX. Unfortunately, nearly 50%of women are unresponsive to anti-ischemic medications when chest pain is caused by CSX [49].

(4) Statins

Statins are one kind of lipid-lowering medications, working by inhibiting the enzyme HMG-CoA reductase required for cholesterol synthesis. Statins can improve endothelial cell function, increase activation of the vasodilator nitric oxide, decrease the vasoconstrictor endothelin-1, improve microvascular vessel tone, decrease inflammation, lower CRP levels, and reduce blood viscosity. In a well-controlled study, 40 patients receiving pravastatin 40 mg daily for 3 months experienced only a mild reduction in cholesterol levels, but had significant improvement in preventing exercise-induced ST segment changes and endothelial cell function [63]. Fábián E reported the chronic statin therapy exerted beneficial effects both on systemic and coronary endothelial function in hypercholesterolemic patients with CSX [75-76].

(5) Angiotensin-Converting Enzyme Inhibitors

Angiotensin-converting enzyme inhibitors (ACE inhibitors) are also important in the treatment of CSX. ACE converts angiotensin I into angiotensin II, a potent vasoconstrictor that increases blood pressure. ACE inhibitors block the conversion and lower blood pressure. In CSX, angiotensin II also causes endothelial cell dysfunction and destroys the vasodilator nitric oxide [63]. Nalbantgil I thought Cilazapril exerted a beneficial therapeutic effect in cases with CSX and the possible mechanism may be a modulation of coronary tone at the microcirculation level [77]. Ozçelik F investigated the anti-ischemic and antianginal effects of nisoldipine (NIS) and ramipril (RAM)in patients with CSX, and observed that 10 mg NIS and 2.5 mg RAM daily had similar anti-ischemic and antianginal effects in patients with syndrome X[78]. New study showed the improvements of various aspects in CSX patients by ACE inhibitors, including endothelial cell function, exercise duration, and exercise-induced ST segment changes [79].

Statin and ACE inhibitor combination therapy is also effective for CSX. A combination of atorvastatin 40 mg and ramipril 10 mg daily showed improved quality of life and endothelial cell function when compared with placebo in a 6-month trial [80].

(6) Estrogen Replacement

As we have known, of the patients with CSX, 60%-70% are women and 60% are postmenopausal women. Estrogen deficiency is a highly suspected contributing factor of CSX. Estrogen can oppose the constricting effect of endothelin-1 and increase coronary blood flow. In addition, estrogen may help CSX patients through analgesic properties affecting the antinociceptive system of the brain. When estrogen level is high, the brain reacts by releasing endorphins that suppress pain signals [81]. Rosano GM found estrogen replacement reduced the frequency of chest pain and ameliorated symptoms in postmenopausal women with syndrome X [82]. Assali AR concluded that transdermal estrogen therapy increased insulin sensitivity in postmenopausal women with CSX. However, this effect was unrelated to the beneficial anti-ischemic effects of estrogen on exercise duration [83].

Although estrogen appears to improve symptoms in some patients with CSX, it is not recommended and remains controversial for the treatment of chronic health conditions [63]. Because estrogen has been associated with an increased risk of endometrial and breast cancer, coronary events, stroke, venous thromboembolism and cholecystitis [81].

(7) Other Medications

The CSX patients with obvious psychological abnormalities can take antidepressants, and (or) anti-anxiety drugs moderately(such as imipramine) [63]. In addition, aminophylline [84-85], L-arginine [70], and analgesics [74] could also be chosen cautiously for the patients with syndrome X in clinical practice.

2. Non-Drug Treatment

(1) Neurostimulation and Spinal Cord Stimulation

Neurostimulation, also named as transcutaneous electrical nerve stimulation (TENS), involves sending low voltage electrical impulses through the skin. Electrical stimulation may alter the way of pain signals to relay to the brain and has been regarded as an effective treatment for many chronic pain conditions such as those with CSX [63].

When TENS therapy is contraindicated, such as when skin irritation from external electrode placement occurs, spinal cord stimulators (SCS) become an option for chronic and refractory pain treatment [65]. Recently, many studies had been carried out to prove that SCS had beneficial effects to the patients with CSX who presented with refractory angina episodes by delaying the onset of chest pain, ST segment changes, and exercise intolerance. In addition, SCS was shown to be able to restore habituation to peripheral pain stimuli. This effect might contribute to restore the ability of CSX patients to better tolerate cardiac pain [86-89].

(2) Psychological Interventions

Some CSX patients have obvious psychological disorders, including anxiety, depression, and panic disorders. Psychological interventions such as relaxation therapy, hyperventilation control, and behavioral therapy through talking and counseling may provide help to relieve chest pain [90]. The CSX patients, especially female ones, can benefit from physical training in terms of exercise capacity and quality of life and from relaxation therapy in terms of quality of life [91].

(3) Enhanced External Counterpulsation

Enhanced external counterpulsation (EECP) has been utilized in the treatment for coronary heart disease, myocardial infarction, stroke and other cardiovascular and cerebrovascular diseases. Recently, Kronhaus KD found EECP also may be an effective and durable treatment by improving endothelial function for CSX. In the study, EECP was used to treat 30 patients with refractory angina due to CSX, with an initial improvement in CCS angina class (3.57 to 1.43; p<0.001) and regional ischemia in all treated patients. At a mean of 11.9 months follow-up, 87% of patients had sustained improvement in angina and were without MACE [92].

By now, there have been a variety of clinical drugs and means can be utilized in the treatment for CSX. However, the unclear pathogenesis of the disease directly impact on the clinical efficacy. Most current treatment could just relieve symptoms, such as chest pain, and not be good to improve the quality of life greatly or even cure the disease completely. Therefore, more effective methods and means still need to be explored for the treatment of CSX.

Section 4 The TCM Studies on CSX

There is no such exact concept like CSX in TCM, but most scholars hold that it belongs to the category of chest impediment and heart pain. From TCM point of view, some experts have done lots of useful tries on the diagnosis and treatment of CSX and proved that TCM has a certain efficacy advantage for the CSX patients. For their different experience and research, the experts reported the different TCM differentiation syndromes and treatment methods. The reports on CSX are as follows.

1. The Summary of TCM Studies n CSX

(1) Treatment Based on TCM Syndrome Differentiation

Zhang MZ reported that the majority of the 20 observed patients with CSX belonged to the TCM syndrome of deficiency in origin and excess in superficiality, especially *Qi* deficiency and blood stasis syndrome. The treatment based on the syndrome differentiation achieved the improvement of symptoms and quality of life[93]. Xu LJ believed the treatment of activating blood flow and removing blood stasis could reduce the plasma concentrations of endothelin-1 and protect endothelial function [94]. Lin N applied *Qi* boosting and *Yang* warming method to 11 CSX cases and got good clinical effect [95]. Zhang XY treated 48 CSX patients by soothing liver and regulating *Qi* method integrated with some western medicine, the clinical efficacy was satisfactory [96]. Wu HL also observed the good therapeutic effect on the method of regulating the spleen to protect the heart in treating myocardial microvascular lesion [97].

(2) Treatment by TCM Classical Formulae

Zhou XH applied *Xuefuzhuyu* decoction for the treatment of 30 CSX cases not only could improve the main symptoms, such as chest pain, but also be helpful to restore ST segment depression on ECG [98]. Zhang XH reported, compared with the effects of isosorbide dinitrate and diltiazem, *Taohongsiwu* decoction to treat 20 patients with CSX showed more obvious effect[99]. Zhao XD applied *Guizhi* decoction associated with *Sinisan* for the treatment of CSX and also achieved obvious clinical efficacy [100].

(3) Treatment with Chinese Patent Medicine

Many researches showed *Tongxinluo* capsule for CSX could relieve angina pectoris, improve ST segment depression on ECG, decrease plasma endothelin-1 concentration and protect endothelial function[101-104]. Wang LW proved *Xuefuzhuyu* capsule could effectively improve CSX patients' the clinical symptoms[105]. Li B observed the efficacy of Heart-protecting Musk pill on CSX patients and found it could significantly alleviate the symptoms of angina pectoris and improve exercise tolerance in patients [106]. Niu TF reported *Xinxuean* granula had a good therapeutic effect for the 30 CSX cases [107]. Li JJ found that *Xuezhikang* could modify endothelin-1 (ET-1), interleukin-6 (IL-6), high-sensitivity C-reactive protein (hs-CRP) and exercise-induced ischemia in CSX patients[108].

2. Our Studies on the TCM Syndrome Patterns and Treatment For CSX

Study 1. Analysis of TCM Syndrome and Pathogenesis Of 12 Patients With CSX
 A total of 12 CSX patients were enrolled, all inpatients from the Cardiovascular Department of the First Teaching Hospital of Tianjin University of TCM from March 2003 to July 2004, their ages ranged form 46 to 66 years old, including 5 men and 7 women. The results were as follows [109].

(1) Analysis of TCM Symptoms
 The main manifestations of 12 CSX patients included serious chest pain, even worse when exercise, chest stuffiness, short breath, palpitations, dark purple tongue with ecchymosis or stasis point, hypertrophy of tongue body, stringy and thready pulse or stopped pulse, and so on. Besides the TCM symptoms above, 5 of them had the mental and physical fatigue, lazy words, irritability, red tongue, or teeth-printed tongue.

(2) Analysis of TCM Pathogenesis
 Chest pain and chest stuffiness, likely to be caused or aggravated when angry or depressed, were the manifestations of *Qi* stagnation. Dark purple tongue with ecchymosis or stasis point, stringy-taut and thready pulse or stopped pulse were the manifestations of blood stasis. In a word, the main TCM pathogenesis of CSX was *Qi* stagnation and blood stasis. Besides, the additional symptoms in 5 patients were due to *Qi* and *Yin* deficiency.

Study 2. Analysis of the TCM Syndrome Patterns of 51 Cases with CSX

The above study[109] had explained the TCM syndrome and pathogenesis characteristics of CSX systematically. However, its analysis on the TCM syndrome patterns of CSX was not enough clear and detailed. On its basis, we summarized the distribution characteristics of the TCM syndrome patterns of 51 CSX patients, all inpatients from the Cardiovascular Department of the First Teaching Hospital of Tianjin University of TCM from March 2003 to January 2006. Their ages ranged form 35 to 71, which included 11 men and 40 women. The results were as follows [110].

Table 1. Analysis of TCM Symptoms Frequency

Symptom	n	Frequency (%)
Chest pain	46	90.2
Chest stuffiness	44	86.3
Abdominal distention	36	70.6
Emotional depression	31	60.8
Sticky mouth	26	51.0
Mental and physical Fatigue	21	41.2
Short breath	20	39.2
Palpitations	19	37.3
Dizziness	18	35.3
Irritability	13	25.5
Anorexia	13	25.5
Fat body	12	23.5
Spontaneous Perspiration	11	21.6
Lazy words	10	19.6
Dry stool	8	15.7
Looking without gloss	6	11.8
Insomnia dream	6	11.8
Thin stool	4	7.8
Tinnitus	4	7.8
Dry mouth	3	5.9
Night sweat	2	3.9
Easy cold	1	2.0
Vexing heat	1	2.0
Forgetful	1	2.0

(1) Analysis of TCM Symptoms Frequency

The most of CSX patients suffered from chest pain (90.2%), chest stuffiness (86.3%), abdominal distention (70.6%), and emotional depression (60.8%). Besides, mental and physical fatigue (41.2%), spontaneous perspiration (21.6%), lazy words (19.6%), looking without gloss(11.8%) and other symptoms could also be seen in clinical practice. (Table 1)

(2) Analysis of the Manifestations of Tongue and Pulse

In 51 patients, there were 25 cases (49%) with dark purple tongue or tongue with petechia, 20 (39.2%) with greasy coating; 19 (37.3%) with stringy-taut pulse , 9 (17.6%) with slippery pulse, and 7 (13.7%) with hesitant pulse. The results of analysis clearly showed that Qi stagnation, phlegm retention and blood stasis were the primary TCM pathogenesis for CSX.

(3) Analysis of TCM Syndrome Patterns Distribution

Based on the statistics and classification of clinical symptoms and the manifestations of tongue and pulse for 51 cases, we had summarized the TCM syndrome patterns distribution of CSX. The results showed that chest pain, chest stuffiness and abdominal distention were the most common manifestations of CSX. Meanwhile, emotional depression and irritability were also the main manifestations. The results suggested that Qi stagnation, phlegm retention and blood stasis were the primary TCM syndrome patterns for CSX. As the development of disease, we also could see Qi deficiency and Yin deficiency in clinical practice. The most of 51 cases (34 cases, 66.7%) were characteristic with the three syndrome factors (Qi stagnation, phlegm retention and blood stasis) at the same time, belonged to simple excess syndrome. There were 17 cases (33.3%) with Qi stagnation, Phlegm retention and blood stasis, as well as deficient syndrome, including Qi deficiency, Yin deficiency, Qi and Yin both deficiency, belonged to integrated deficient and excess syndrome.

The results of completed studies[109-110] suggested that, chest pain and chest stuffiness were the main manifestations of CSX, and Qi stagnation, phlegm retention and blood stasis were the mostly TCM syndrome patterns for CSX. Based on the TCM pathogenesis characteristics of CSX above, Qi-regulating, chest-relaxing and blood-activating therapy was determined as the main TCM treatment method. For evaluating the clinical efficacy of the method in treating CSX patients, We desinged and practiced a randomized controlled trial (RCT) in the following studies.

Study 3. Summary of 32 CSX Patients Treated by *Qi*-Regulating, Chest-Relaxing and Blood-Activating Therapy of TCM

By coin tossing method, totally 51 CSX patients were randomly assigned to the control group(19 cases) and the treatment group(32 cases). In the control group, the patients were treated with conventional western medication, including nitroglycerin injection 5-10 mg diluted by 500ml of 5% glucose for intravenous dripping, 20-30 drops/min, once daily, and if necessary Betaloc 6.25-25 mg, twice daily and/or diltiazem hydrochloride 30 mg, three times per day. In the treatment group, the patients were treated with the same conventional western medication as used in the control one, and the herbal decoction of *Qi*-regulating, chest-relaxing and blood-activating additionally, one dose of which composed of *Radix Bupleuri*10g, *Fructus Aurantii*12g, *Rhizoma Chuanxiong*10g, *Radix Angelicae sinensis*12g, *Pericarpium Trichosanthis*15g, *Bulbus Allii macrostemi*10g, *Radix Salviae miltiorrhizae*15g, *Yunnan Poria*12g, *Rhizoma Atractylodes alba*12g, *Pericarpium Citri reticulatae*12g, *Flos Carthami*15g and *Rhizoma Corydalis*15g.The decoction was prepared by water doused and boiled down to about 300ml, and taken 150ml once, twice a day. The treatment course was 14 days.

We had observed the conditions of angina pectoris, TCM clinical symptoms, TCM syndrome and treadmill exercise test before and after treatment, and the results were as follows [111].

(1) Clinical Efficacy on Angina Pectoris

In the treatment group, the clinical efficacy on angina pectoris in 19 cases was judged as markedly effective, 8 as effective, the total effective rate was 81.2%; while in the control one, in 7 cases as markedly effective, 3 as effective, and the total effective rate was 52.6%. The total effective rate in the former was obviously better than that in the latter($P<0.05$).

**Table 2. Comparison of the Effect on Main Symptoms
between Groups($\bar{x} \pm s$)**

Symptom	Control group (n=19)		Treatment group (n=32)	
	BT	AT	BT	AT
Chest pain	2.31±0.01	1.72±0.54△	2.42±0.01	1.21±0.58▲☆
Chest stuffiness	2.02±0.69	1.54±0.61△	2.22±0.67	1.04±0.65▲☆
Abdominal distention	1.84±0.52	1.63±0.69	1.94±0.61	1.45±0.62△
Fidgetiness	1.92±0.83	1.43±0.82△	2.14±0.75	1.67±0.55△
Palpitation	1.93±0.64	1.63±0.66	1.74±0.68	0.68±0.76▲☆

Notes: △P<0.05, ▲P<0.01, compared with before treatment; ☆P<0.05, compared with the control group after treatment; BT: before treatment; AT: after treatment.

(2) Effect on Main Symptoms

As shown in Table 2, the effect on chest pain, chest stuffiness, abdominal distention, fidgetiness and palpitation in the treatment group was significantly better than that before treatment (P<0.05 or P<0.01), while in the control group improvement was only shown on chest pain, chest stuffiness and fidgetiness (P<0.05). The comparison between two groups showed that the effect on chest pain, chest stuffiness and palpitation in the treatment group was significantly better than that on those in the control group(P<0.05), while the effects on abdominal distention and fidgetiness were insignificantly different between the two groups (P>0.05).

(3) Effect on TCM Syndrome

As shown in Table 3, in the treatment group 15 cases were markedly effective, 12 effective and the total effective rate was 84.4%; while in the control one, 6 cases were markedly effective, 5 effective and the total effective rate was 57.9%. The total effective rate on TCM syndrome in the treatment group was obviously better than that in the control one(P<0.05).

Table 3. Comparison of the Effect on TCM Syndrome in the Two Groups(Case)

Effect	Control group (n=19)	Treatment group (n=32)
Markedly effective	6	15
Effective	5	12
Ineffective	8	5
Aggravated	0	0
Total effective (%)	57.9	84.4$^{☆}$

Notes: $^{☆}$P<0.05, compared with the control group.

(4) Effect on Treadmill Exercise Test

Before treatment, treadmill exercise test was carried out on 51 patients and it was rechecked after treatment in 35 patients (22 in the Treatment group and 13 in the control one). The results were listed in detail in Table 4.

The outcome of treadmill exercise test showed the maximal metabolic equivalent (Max MET) and the time of angina onset and ST segment depression by 0.1 mV were obviously improved after treatment in both groups. However, the improvement in the treatment group was significantly better than that in the control one (P<0.05).

Table 4. Comparison of the Effect on Treadmill Exercise Test between Groups($\bar{x} \pm s$)

Items	Control group		Treatment group	
	BT (n=19)	AT(n=13)	BT (n=32)	AT (n=22)
Item one (Mets)	5.31±1.08	6.02±0.84$^{△}$	5.57±2.12	7.33±0.96$^{▲☆}$
Item two (s)	222±99.63	286±76.53$^{△}$	245±60.91	360.67±64.77$^{▲☆}$

Notes: $^{△}$P<0.05, $^{▲}$P<0.01, compared with before treatment; $^{☆}$P<0.05, compared with the control group after treatment; Item one : Maximal metabolic equivalent; Item two: Time of angina onset and ST segment depressed by 0.1 mV; BT: before treatment; AT: after treatment.

(5)Adverse Reactions and Drug Safety Situation

In the course of treatment, one patient of the control group was flustered after sublingual nitroglycerin, and the symptoms disappeared on his own for a moment; 32 patients of the Treatment group had no obvious adverse reactions. The blood, urine, and liver and renal functions tests of two groups showed no obviously abnormal changes before and after treatment.

Study 4. Further RCT Study on *Qi*-Regulating, Chest-Relaxing and Blood-Activating Therapy for CSX

A total of 55 CSX patients, 18 to 74 years old, 8 male and 47 female, were enrolled. All of them were inpatients from the Cardiovascular Department of the First Teaching Hospital of Tianjin University of TCM from July 2006 to August 2007, in line with the TCM syndrome standards of *Qi* stagnation, phlegm retention and blood stasis. By random number table method, all cases were randomly assigned to the control group (27 cases) and the treatment one (28 cases). The patients in the control group were treated with conventional western medication, including nitroglycerin injection 5-10 mg diluted by 500ml of 5% glucose for intravenous dripping, 20-30 drops/min, once daily, and if necessary Betaloc 6.25-12.5mg, twice daily, and/or diltiazem hydrochloride 30 mg, and/or monroe hydrochloride 5-10 mg, once daily. The patients in the treatment one were treated with the same medication as used in the control one, and the herbal decoction of *Qi*-regulating, Chest-relaxing and Blood-activating additionally, one dose of which composed of *Radix Bupleuri*10g, *Fructus Aurantii*12g, *Melon wilt Paper*15g, *Rhizoma Chuanxiong*10g, *Radix Angelicae sinensis*12g, *Bulbus Allii macrostemi*10g, *Radix Salviae miltiorrhizae*15g, *Yunnan Poria*12g, *Pericarpium Citri reticulatae*12g, *Rhizoma Atractylodis Macrocephalae*12g, *Rhzoma Corydalis* 15g, *Carthamus tinctorius* 15g. The decoction was prepared by decocting crude drugs with water, boiled down to about 300ml, and taken 150ml once, twice a day. The treatment course was 14 days.

We had observed the conditions of angina pectoris, TCM syndrome, electrocardiogram, treadmill exercise test, and the levels of ET-l, NO, and hs-CRP before and after treatment. The results were as follows [112].

(1) Clinical Efficacy on Angina Pectoris

As shown in Table 5, in the treatment group, the clinical efficacy on angina pectoris in 17 cases was judged as markedly effective, 6 as effective, the total effective rate was 82.14%; While in the control one, in 12 cases as markedly effective, 3 as effective, and the total effective rate was 55.56%. The total effective rate in the former was obviously better than that in the latter(P<0.05).

(2) Effect on TCM Syndrome

As shown in Table 6, the effect on TCM syndrome of 13 cases were judged as markedly effective, 11 effective, and the total effective rate was 82.14% in the Treatment group; While 8 cases as markedly effective, 7 effective, and the total effective rate was 55.56% in the control one. The total effective rate on TCM syndrome in the treatment group was obviously better than that in the control one (P<0.05).

Table 5. Comparison of the Effect on Angina Pectoris (Case)

Effect	Control group (n=27)	Treatment group (n=28)
Markedly effective	12	17
Effective	3	6
Ineffective	12	5
Aggravated	0	0
Total effective (%)	55.56	82.14*

Notes: *P<0.05, compared with the control group.

Table 6. Comparison of the Effect on TCM Syndrome in the Two Groups(Case)

Effect	Control group (n=27)	Treatment group (n=28)
Markedly effective	8	13
Effective	7	11
Ineffective	12	4
Aggravated	0	0
Total effective (%)	55.56	82.14*

Notes: *P<0.05, compared with the control group.

(3) Effect on Electrocardiogram

As shown in Table 7, the effect on electrocardiogram of 7 cases proved to be markedly effective, 8 effective, and the total effective rate was 53.57% in the treatment group; While 5 cases proved it to be markedly effective, 8 effective, and the total effective rate was 48.15% in the control one. There was no significant difference of the total effective rate on electrocardiogram between the Treatment group and the control group($P > 0.05$).

Before treatment, treadmill exercise test was carried out on 55 patients and it was rechecked after treatment in 40 patients (18 in the treatment group and 22 in the control one). The results were listed in detail in Table 8.

Table 7. Comparison of the Effect on Electrocardiogram in the Two Groups(Case)

Effect	Control group (n=27)	Treatment group (n=28)
Markedly effective	5	7
Effective	8	8
Ineffective	14	13
Aggravated	0	0
Total effective (%)	48.15	53.57

Table 8. Comparison of the Effect on Treadmill Exercise Test between Groups($\overline{x} \pm s$)

Items	Control group		Treatment group	
	BT (n=27)	AT(n=22)	BT (n=28)	AT (n=18)
Item one (Mets)	5.56±1.24	6.21±0.72△	5.86±1.76	7.24±0.87△☆
Item two (s)	243±78.76	295±65.73△	248±80.81	347±71.66△☆
Item three (mm)	7.5±2.1	6.2±1.7△	7.9±2.3	5.3±1.8△☆

Notes: △$P<0.05$, compared with before treatment; ☆$P<0.05$, compared with the control group after treatment; Item one: Maximal metabolic equivalent; Item two: Exercise duration; Item three: ST segment depressed after exercise; BT: before treatment; AT: after treatment.

(4) Effect on Treadmill Exercise Test

The outcome of treadmill exercise test showed the maximal metabolic equivalent, exercise duration and ST segment depression after exercise were obviously improved after treatment in both groups (P<0.05). However, the improvement in the treatment group was better than that in the control one (P<0.05). The outcome showed that the herbal decoction of Qi-regulating, chest-relaxing and blood-activating could improve patients' exercise tolerance.

(5) Effect on the Levels of ET-L, NO, and Hs-CRP

Before treatment, the tests of ET-l, NO, and hs-CRP were carried out on 55 patients and they were rechecked after treatment in 46 patients (25 in the Treatment group and 21 in the control one). The results were listed in detail in Table 9.

The outcome of tests showed the levels of ET-l, NO, and hs-CRP were obviously improved after treatment in both groups (P<0.05). Meanwhile, the improvement in the treatment group was better than that in the control one (P<0.05). The outcome proved that the herbal decoction of Qi-regulating, chest-relaxing and blood-activating could inhibit inflammatory response of vascular wall and protect the function of vascular endothelial cell.

Table 9. Comparison of the Effect on ET-l, NO, and hs-CRP Test between Groups($\overline{x} \pm s$)

Items	Control group BT (n=27)	AT(n=22)	Treatment group BT (n=28)	AT (n=18)
ET-1 (ng/L)	99.64±12.61	64.06±15.45Δ	94.97±10.24	50.01±13.20 Δ☆
NO (umol/L)	45.41±5.91	54.69±4.62 Δ	46.07±5.83	62.34±5.60Δ ☆
hs-CRP (mg/L)	3.47±0.24	2.31±0.28 Δ	3.48±0.25	1.80±0.17Δ ☆

Notes: ΔP<0.05, compared with before treatment; ☆P<0.05, compared with the control group after treatment; BT: before treatment; AT: after treatment.

(6) Security Analysis

In the course of treatment, two groups of patients had no obvious adverse reactions found. The blood, urine, and liver and renal functions tests of two groups showed no obviously abnormal changes before and after treatment.

Our studies[109-112] showed that CSX as a kind of clinical syndrome could be found in different age, and women were more likely to affect the disease than men. From TCM's point of view, the etiology of CSX was related to liver, the diseased part was in heart, and the spleen dysfunction also involved to it. *Qi* stagnation, phlegm retention and blood stasis were determined as the basic TCM pathogenesis, and heart meridian blocking was the pathological results. We have summarized that the TCM syndrome of *Qi* stagnation, phlegm retention and blood stasis was the basic syndrome of CSX throughout the whole course of the disease. As a result, we took *Qi*-regulating, chest-relaxing and blood-activating as the main TCM treatment method and treated CSX patients with *Qi*-regulating, chest-relaxing and blood-activating therapy and integrated with some western medicine. The results of RCT showed that, on the basis of conventional western medication, *Qi*-regulating, chest-relaxing and blood-activating therapy had better clinical efficacy than simple conventional western medication alone. *Qi*-regulating, chest-relaxing and blood-activating therapy could reduce the frequency and degree of the occurrence of angina, improve patients' TCM syndromes and exercise tolerance. Meanwhile, the treatment method could inhibit inflammatory response of vascular wall and protect the function of vascular endothelial cell.

In a word, TCM had a certain efficacy advantage in improving clinical syndrome and quality of life for the CSX patients. The traditional Chinese medicine provided a new effective approach for the prevention and treatment of CSX. However, the current TCM syndrome analysis on CSX was still not enough in-depth, some long-term, multi-centers, randomized controlled trials with large sample are still required for evaluating the clinical efficacy and safety of TCM therapies.

Section 5 Prognosis of CSX

Without a definitive etiology, it is difficult to predict the prognosis of CSX. Therefore, the prognosis of CSX is not quite clear at present. Early studies suggested an good prognosis for survival in CSX with preserved left ventricular function when compared with other types of cardiovascular events

[64]. But now, there are newer data to indicate more than 40% of the CSX patients re-admitted to hospital because of chest pain, 30% again coronary angiography in 5 years [113]. Approximately 50% of sufferers said that their lives were significantly disabled, 50% were or became unemployed, and 75% continued to see a physician for CSX symptoms [90]. CSX may severely affect the quality of life, and almost half of patients continue to have disabling pain resistant to anti-ischemic medications after medical intervention [49]. In addition, compared with the general population, these patients have higher incidence rates of myocardial infarction and stroke [114]. When compared with obstructive coronary heart disease, the overall cardiovascular event rate for CSX is relatively low. However, women with CSX experience myocardial infarction, congestive heart failure, stroke, and death at more than double the rate of an average woman in the same age [49].

Conclusion

CSX patients have typical chest pain, with ST segment changes and normal coronary angiography. The diagnostic criteria look simple, and the triad of clinical features should be existing at the same time. Although coronary angiograms normal, it is incorrect to tell patients there is nothing wrong with their heart when they meet the diagnostic criteria for CSX.

The pathogenesis of CSX is complicated, resulting from a variety of pathogenic factors, unfortunately, not quite clear at present. The pathogenesis studies of CSX still need to be further explored and clarifying its pathogenesis can help to improve the treatment level of the disease. Current studies suggest coronary endothelial cell dysfunction is the leading cause of CSX and plays very important role in the pathogenesis of CSX. Therefore, intervention with medications, such as statins, ACE inhibitors and estrogen replacement, are being used to correct endothelial cell dysfunction. In addition, anti-ischemic medications can help some patients achieve pain relief. Additionally, Patients with CSX may also be referred to psychological services for treatment, which can be effective. When pain is intractable or refractory, neurostimulation and spinal cord stimulation may be beneficial. Enhanced external counterpulsation, a kind of new treatment for CSX, also can be chosen when necessary. If causative pathogenic factors are identified, the treatment must be individualized. However, because of the unclear pathogenesis, common medications and therapies sometimes can not well improve the symptoms and quality of life in clinical practice.

Traditional Chinese medicine is the unique wealth of china, and has spread for thousands of years. There are different angles and aspects from the western medicine to recognize the pathogenesis and treatment for CSX. From TCM's point of view, Chinese medical experts have done some useful tries on the diagnosis and treatment of CSX and proved that TCM has a certain efficacy advantage for the treatment of CSX patients. Therefore, we treat CSX patients with Qi-regulating, chest-relaxing and blood-activating therapy, integrated with some western medicine. On the basis of conventional western medication, Qi-regulating, chest-relaxing and blood-activating therapy had better clinical efficacy than simple conventional western medication alone. The traditional Chinese medicine may provide a kind of new effective approach for the prevention and treatment of CSX.

References

[1] Likoff, W; Seagal, BL; Kasparin H. Paradox of normal elective coronary arteriogram in patients considered to have unmistakable coronary hert disease [J]. *N. Eng. J. Med.,* 1967, 276(5): 1063.

[2] Kemp, HG. Left ventricular function in patients with the anginal syndrome and normal coronary arteriograms [J]. *Am. J. Cardiol.,* 1976, 32(5): 375.

[3] Cannon, RO; Epstein, SE. "Microvascular angina" as a cause of chest pain with angiographically normal coronary arteries [J]. *Am. J. Cardio,* 1988, 61(15):1338-1343.

[4] Kaski, JC. Chest Pain with Normal Coronary Angiograms: Pathogenesis, Diagnosis and Management [M]. London, UK: Kluwer Academic Publishers, 1999.

[5] Goel, PK; Gupta, SK; Agarwal, A; et al. Slow coronary flow: a distinct angiographic subgroup in syndrome X [J]. *Angiology,* 2001, 52(8): 507-514.

[6] Fragasso, G; Chierchia, SL; Arioli, F; et al. Coronary slow-flow causing transient myocardial hypoperfusion in patients with cardiac syndrome X: long-term clinical and functional prognosis [J]. *Int. J. Cardiol.,* 2009, 137 (2): 137-144.

[7] Jiang, JQ; Chen, L; Lin, QR; et al. The diagnostic value of dipyridamole (201)Tl-SPECT myocardial imaging and exercise myocardial (99)Tc(m)-MIBI-SPECT imaging on detecting cardiac syndrome X [J]. *Chinese Journal Of Cardiovascular Diseases,*2009 ,37 (7): 615-617.

[8]   Lanza, GA; Buffon, A; Sestito, A; et al. Relation between stress-induced myocardial perfusion defects on cardiovascular magnetic resonance and coronary microvascular dysfunction in patients with cardiac syndrome X [J]. *J. Am. Coll. Cardiol*,2008,51 (4): 466-472.

[9]   Cotrim, C; Almeida, AG; Carrageta, M. Exercise-induced intra-ventricular gradients as a frequent potential cause of myocardial ischemia in cardiac syndrome X patients [J]. *Cardiovasc. Ultrasound*, 2008, 6: 3.

[10]   Galuto, L; Sestito, A; Barchetta, S; et al. Noninvasive evaluation of flow reserve in the leftanterior descending coronary artery in patientswith cardiac syndrome X [J]. *Am. J. Cardio.*, 2007, 99(10): 1378-1383.

[11]   Saghari, M; Assadi, M; Eftekhari,M; et al. Frequency and severity of myocardial perfusion abnormalities using Tc-99mMIBISPECT in cardiac syndrome X [J]. *BMC Nucl.Med.*, 2006, 6: 1.

[12]   Cavusoglu, Y; Entok, E; Timuralp, B; et al. Regional distribution and extent of perfusion abnormalities, and the lung to heart uptake ratios during exercise thallium-201 SPECT imaging in patients with cardiac syndrome X [J]. *Can .J. Cardio.*, 2005, 21(1): 57.

[13]   Qian, JY; Ge, JB; Fan,B; et al. Identification of syndromeX using intravascularul trasound imaging and Doppler flow mapping [J].*Chin. Med. J.* (Engl), 2004, 117(4): 521-527.

[14]   Panting, JR; Gatehouse, PD; Yang, GZ; et al. Abnormal subendocardial perfusion in cardiac syndrome X detected by cardiovascular magnetic resonance imaging [J].*N. Engl. J. Med.*, 2002, 346(25): 1948-1953.

[15]   Reis, SE; Holubkov, R. Coronary microvascular dysfunction is highly prevalent in women with chest pain in the absence of coronary artery disease: results from the NHLBIWISE study [J]. *Am. Heart J.*, 2001, 141(5): 735-741.

[16]   Zhang, P; Jiang, JQ. Research on the pathogenesis of CSX - endothelial dysfunction [J]. *Chinese Journal of Cardiovascular Rehabilitation Medicine*, 2007, 16(2): 195-197.

[17]   Wang, XL; Mao, JY; Wang, HH. Research on Cardiac Syndrome X and related cytokines [J]. *Chinese Journal of Cardiovascular Review*, 2007, 5(5): 372.

[18]   Shmilovich, H; Deutsch, V; Roth, A;et al. Circulating endothelial progenitor cells in patients with cardiac syndrome X [J]. *Heart*,2007 ,93 (9): 1071-1076.

[19] Huang, PH; Chen, YH; Chen, YL; et al. Vascular endothelial function and circulating endothelial progenitor cells in patients with cardiac syndrome X.[J]. *Heart*, 2007, 93 (9): 1064-1070.

[20] Goon, PK; Lip, GY. Endothelial progenitor cells, endothelial cell dysfunction and much more: observations from cardiac syndrome X.[J]. *Heart*, 2007, 93 (9): 1020-1021.

[21] Gil-Ortega, I; Marzoa, Rivas R; Ríos, Vázquez R; et al. Role of inflammation and endothelial dysfunction in the pathogenesis of cardiac syndrome X [J]. *Future Cardiol.,* 2006 , 2 (1): 63-73.

[22] Ding, RJ; Lv, ZX; Zhou, XC; et al. Analysis of changes between endothelin, nitric oxide and ET-1/NO ratio during exercise in patients with cardiac syndrome X [J]. *Journal of Elinical Research*,2005,22(6):741-743.

[23] Wu, YT; Gao, YC; Cao, SJ; et al. Changes of plasma levels of nitrie oxide and fuaction of endothelium dependent vasodilation in the patients with X syndrome [J]. *Journal of Clinical Cardiology,* 2004, 20: 195-196.

[24] Kolasinska-Kloch, W; Lesniak, W; Kiec-Wilk, B; et al. Biochemical parameters of endothelial dysfunction in cardiological syndrome X [J]. *Scand. J. Clin. Lab. Invest.,* 2002, 62(1): 7-13.

[25] Gewaltig, MT; Kojda, G. Vaso protection by nitric oxide: mechanisms and therapeutic potential [J].*Cardiovasc. Res.,* 2002, 55(2): 250-260.

[26] Zhang, WF; Chen, JZ; Xu, Q; et al. Changes of plasma endothelin levels in coronary circulation in patients with syndrome X [J]. *Chinese Journal of Cardiology*, 2001, 29(3): 158-159.

[27] Hu, ZT; Yang, JG; Wang, X; et al. A study on insulin resistance and the relationship between insulin resistance and endothelin or nitric oxide in patients with cardiological syndrome X [J]. *Journal of Clinical Cardiology*,2001,17(4):170-172.

[28] Suwaidi, JA; Hamasaki, S; Higano,ST; et al. Long-term follow up of patients with mild coronary artery disease and endothelialdys function [J]. *Circulation*, 2000, 101(9): 948-954.

[29] Rosen, SD; Paulesu, E; W ise, RJS; et al. Central neural contribution to the perception of chest pain in cardiac syndromeX [J]. *Heart,* 2002, 87(6): 513-519.

[30] Valeriani, M; Sestito, A; Pera, DL; et al. Abnormal corticalpain processing in patients with cardiac syndromeX [J]. *Eur. Heart J.,* 2005, 26(10): 975-982.

[31] Lanza, GA; Giordano, AG; Pristipino, C; et al. Abnormal cardiac adrenergic nerve function in patients with syndrome X detected by [123I] metaiodobenzylguanidine myocardial scintigraphy [J]. *Circulation*, 1997, 96(3): 821-826.

[32] Chauhan, A; Mullins, PA; Thuraisingham, SI; et al. Abnormal cardiac pain perception in syndromeX [J. *J. Am. Coll. Cardio.*, 1994, 24: 329-335.

[33] Assadi, M; Saghari, M; Ebrahimi, A;et al. The relation between Helicobacter pylori infection and cardiac syndrome X: A preliminary study [J]. *Int. J. Cardiol.*, 2009 ,134 (3): 124-125.

[34] Eroglu, S; Elif-Sade, L; Yildirir, A; et al. Serum levels of C-reactive protein and uric acid in patients with cardiac syndrome X [J]. *Acta Cardiol.*, 2009, 64 (2): 207-211.

[35] Rasmi, Y; Raeisi, S. Possible role of Helicobacter pylori infection via microvascular dysfunction in cardiac syndrome X [J]. *Cardiol. J.*, 2009, 16 (6): 585-587.

[36] Atmaca, Y; Ozdol, C; Turhan, S; et al. The association of elevated white blood cell count and C-reactive protein with endothelial dysfunction in cardiac syndrome X [J]. *Acta Cardiol.*, 2008, 63 (6): 723-728.

[37] Dabek, J; Kulach, A; Wilzok, T; et al. Transcriptional activity of genes encoding interferon gamma (IFN gamma) and its receptor assessed in peripheral blood mononuclear cells in patients with cardiac syndrome X [J]. *Inflammation*, 2007, 30: 125-129.

[38] Song, YH; Dai, YG; Cai, LA. Association of helicobacter pylori infection with cardiac syndrome X [J]. *Chinese Journal of Cardiovascular Review*, 2007, 5 (6): 456-458.

[39] Eskandarian, R; Malek, M; Mousavi, SH; et al. Association of Helicobacter pylori infection with cardiac syndrome X [J]. *Singapore Med .J.*,2006, 47(8): 704-706.

[40] Arroyo, ER; Nadia, M; Pablo, A; et al. Chronic inflammation and inceased arterial stiffness in patients with cardiac syndrome X [J]. *Eur. Heart J.*, 2003, 24(22): 2006-2011.

[41] Tousoulis, D; Davies, GJ; Asimakopoulos, G; et al. Vascular cell adhesion molecule-1 and intercellular adhesion molecule-1 serum level in patients with chest pain and normal coronary arteries (syndrome X) [J] . *Clin. Cardiol.*, 2001, 24: 301-304.

[42] Maseri, A. Women's ischemic syndrome evaluation: current status and future research directions: report of the National Heart, lung and blood institute workshop: October2-4, 2002: perspective: new frontiers in

detection of ischemic heart disease in women [J]. *Circulation,* 2004, 109(6): 662.

[43] Hayward, CS; Kelly, RP; Collins, P; et al. The roles of gender, themenopause and hormone replacement on cardiovascular function [J]. *Cardiovasc. Res.,* 2000, 46: 28-49.

[44] Gilligan, DM; Badar, DM; Panza, JA; et al. Acute vascular effects of oestrogen in postmenopausal women [J]. *Circulation,* 1994, 90: 786-791.

[45] Peters, NS; Milson, I. Benificial effect of treatment with transdermal estradiol-17 β on exercise included angina and ST segment depression in syndrome X [J].*Int. J. Cardiol.,* 2000; 64(2): 13.

[46] Roque, M; Hares, M; Roig, E; et al. Short-term effects of transdermal estrogen replacement therapy on coronary vascular reavtivity in postmenopausal women with angina pectoris and normal results on coronary angiograms [J]. *J. Am. Coll. Cardiol.,* 1998: 31(1): 139.

[47] Vermeltfoort, IA; Raijmakers, PG; Odekerken, DA; et al. Association between anxiety disorder and the extent of ischemia observed in cardiac syndrome X [*J]. J. Nucl. Cardiol.,* 2009, 16 (3): 405-410.

[48] Piegza, M; Pudlo, R; Badura-Brzoza, K; et al. Cardiac syndrome X from a psychosomatic point of view [J]. *Psychiatr. Pol.,* 2008, 42 (2): 229-236.

[49] Johnson, B; Shaw, L; Pepine, C; et al. Persistent chest pain predicts cardiovascular events in women without obstructive coronary artery disease: Results from the NIH-NHLBI-sponsored Women's Ischaemia Syndrome Evaluation (WISE) study. *Eur. Heart J.,* 2006, 27: 1408–1415.

[50] Asbury, EA; Creed, F; Collins, P. Distinct psychosocial differences between women with coronary heart disease and cardiac syndrome X [J].*Eur. Heart J.,* 2004, 25(19): 1695-1701.

[51] Nijher, G; Weinman, J; Bass, C; et al. Chest pain in people with normal coronary anatomy [J]. *BMJ,* 2001, 323:1319.

[52] Sen, N; Poyraz, F; Tavil, Y;et al. Carotid intima-media thickness in patients with cardiac syndrome X and its association with high circulating levels of asymmetric dimethylarginine [J]. Atherosclerosis, 2009, 204 (2): 82-85.

[53] Timurkaynak, T; Balcioglu, S; Arslan, U; et al. Plasma homocysteine level in cardiac syndrome X and its relation with duke treadmill score [J]. *Saudi Med. J.,* 2008, 29 (3): 364-367.

[54] Alroy, S; Preis,M; Barzilai,M; et al. Endothelial cell dysfunction in women with cardiac syndrome X and MTHFR C677T mutation [J]. *Isr. Med. Assoc. J.,* 2007, 653.

[55] Dean, JD; Jones, CJ; Hutchison, SJ; et al. Hyperinsulinaemia and microvascular angina ("syndromeX") [J].*Lancet,* 1991, 337: 456-457.

[56] Botker, HE; Frobert, O; Moller, N; et al. Insulin resistance in cardiac syndrome X and variant angina [J].*Am. Heart J.,* 1997, 134: 229-237.

[57] Cay, S; Biyikoglu, F; Cihan, G; et al. Mean platelet volumein the patients with cardiac syndrome X. *Journal of Thrombosis and Thrombolysis,* 2005, 20(3): 175–178.

[58] Qin, RJ. Clinical hemorheology [M].Beijing: Peking University *Medical. Press.,* 2003:4.

[59] Gur, M; Yildiz, A; Demirbag, R; et al. Increased lymphocyte deoxyribonucleic acid damage in patients with cardiac syndromeX [J]. *Mutat. Res.,* 2007, 617(1-2): 8-15.

[60] Gur, M; Yildiz, A; Demirbag, R; et al. Paraoxonase and arylesterase activities in patients with cardiac syndrome X and their relationship with oxidative stress markers [J]. *Coron. Artery Dis.,* 2007, 18(2): 89-95.

[61] Quyyumi AA . Does acute improvement of endothelial dysfunction in coronary artery disease improve myocardial ischemia? A double – blind comparison of parenteral D-and L-arginine [J]. *JACC,* 1998, 32(4): 904-911.

[62] Liu, QM; Zhou, SH; Zhao, SP. Research on Microvascular Angina [J]. *Foreign Medical Sciences Section of Pathophysiology and Clinical Medicine,*1999, 19(2): 129.

[63] Kaski, JC; Aldama, G; Cosín-Sales, J. Cardiac syndrome X. Diagnosis, pathogenesis and management [J]. *Am. J. Cardiovasc. Drugs,*2004,4 (3):179-94.

[64] Larsen, W; Mandleco, B. Chest pain with angiographic clear coronary arteries: A provider's approach to cardiac syndrome X [J]. *J. Am. Acad. Nurse Pract.,* 2009, 21 (7): 371-376.

[65] Lanza, G. Cardiac syndrome X: Acritical overview and future perspectives [J]. *Heart,* 2007, 93: 159-166.

[66] Hurst, T; Olson, TH; Olson, LE; et al. Cardiac syndrome X and endothelial dysfunction: new concepts in prognosis and treatment [J]. *Am. J. Med.,* 2006, 119 (7): 560-566.

[67] Bugiardini, R; Merz, CN. Angina with''normal''coronary arteries: a changing philosophy [J]. *JAMA,* 2005, 293(4): 477-484.

[68] Lanza, GA; Manzoli, A; Bia, E; et al. Acute effects of nitrates on exercise testing in patients with syndrome X. Clinical and pathophysiological implications [J]. *Circulation*, 1994, 90 (6): 2695-2700.

[69] Radice, M; Giudici, V; Pusineri, E;et al. Different effects of acute administration of aminophylline and nitroglycerin on exercise capacity in patients with syndrome X [J]. *Am. J. Cardiol.*, 1996 ,78 (1): 88-92.

[70] Deng, HQ. Pathogenesis and treatment of Cardiac syndrome X [J]. *South China Journal of Cardiovascular Diseases*, 2008, 14(6): 390-391.

[71] Lanza, GA; Colonna, G; Pasceri, V; et al. Atenolol versus amlodipine versus isosorbide-5-mononitrate on anginal symptoms in syndrome X [J]. *Am. J. Cardiol.*, 1999, 84 (7): 854-856.

[72] Sen, N; Tavil, Y; Erdamar, H; et al. Nebivolol therapy improves endothelial function and increases exercise tolerance in patients with cardiac syndrome X [J]. *Anadolu. Kardiyol. Derg.*, 2009, 9 (5): 371-379.

[73] Erdamar, H; Sen, N; Tavil, Y; et al. The effect of nebivolol treatment on oxidative stress and antioxidant status in patients with cardiac syndrome-X [J]. *Coron. Artery Dis.*, 2009, 20 (3): 238-244.

[74] Bao, ZY; Mao, JL. Diagnosis and therapy of cardiac syndrome X [J]. *Advances in Cardiovascular Diseases*, 2006, 27(3): 298.

[75] Fábián, E; Varga, A. Effect of simvastatin therapy on endothelial function of hypercholesteremic patients with syndrome X [J]. *Orv. Hetil.*, 2002, 143 (36): 2067-2071.

[76] Fábián, E; Varga, A; Picano, E; et al. Effect of simvastatin on endothelial function in cardiac syndrome X patients [J]. *Am. J. Cardiol.*, 2004, 94 (5): 652-655.

[77] Nalbantgil, I; Onder, R; Altintig, A;et al. Therapeutic benefits of cilazapril in patients with syndrome X [J]. *Cardiology*, 1998, 89 (2): 130-133.

[78] Ozçelik, F; Altun, A; Ozbay, G. Antianginal and anti-ischemic effects of nisoldipine and ramipril in patients with syndrome X [J]. *Clin. Cardiol.*, 1999, 22 (5): 361-365.

[79] Arroyo-Espliguero, R; Kaski, J. Microvascular dysfunction in cardiac syndrome X: The role of inflammation [J]. *CMAJ*, 2006, 174(13): 1833–1834.

[80] Pizzi, C; Manfrini, O; Fontana, F; et al. Angiotensin-converting enzyme inhibitorsa nd 3-hydroxy-3-methylglutaryl coenzyme A reductase in cardiac syndrome X[J]. *Circulation*, 2004, 109(1): 53-58.

[81] Kaski, J. Cardiac syndrome X in women: The role of oestrogen deficiency [J]. *Heart*, 2006, 92(Suppl 3): iii5–iii9.

[82] Rosano, GM; Peters, NS; Lefroy, D;et al. 17-beta-Estradiol therapy lessens angina in postmenopausal women with syndrome X [J]. *J. Am. Coll. Cardiol.*, 1996, 28 (6): 1500-1505.

[83] Assali, AR; Jabara, Z; Shafer, Z. Insulin resistance is increased by transdermal estrogen therapy in postmenopausal women with cardiac syndrome X [J]. *Cardiology*, 2001, 95 (1): 31-34.

[84] Yeşildağ, O; Yazici, M; Yilmaz, O; et al. The effect of aminophylline infusion on the exercise capacity in patients with syndrome X [J]. *Acta Cardiol.*, 1999, 54 (6): 335-337.

[85] Elliott, PM; Krzyzowska-Dickinson, K; Calvino, R; et al. Effect of oral aminophylline in patients with angina and normal coronary arteriograms (cardiac syndrome X) [J]. *Heart*, 1997 ,77 (6): 523-526.

[86] Sgueglia, GA; Sestito, A. Spinal cord stimulation: a new form of pain modulatory treatment in cardiac syndrome X [J]. *Am. J. Med.*, 2007, 120 (9): e17.

[87] Sgueglia, GA; Sestito, A; Spinelli, A; et al. Long-term follow-up of patients with cardiac syndrome X treated by spinal cord stimulation [J]. *Heart*, 2007, 93 (5): 591-597.

[88] Sestito, A; Lanza, GA; Le-Pera, D; et al. Spinal cord stimulation normalizes abnormal cortical pain processing in patients with cardiac syndrome X [J]. *Pain*, 2008, 139 (1): 82-89.

[89] Spinelli, A; Lanza, GA; Calcagni, ML; et al. Effect of spinal cord stimulation on cardiac adrenergic nerve function in patients with cardiac syndrome X [J]. *J. Nucl. Cardiol.*, 2008, 15 (6): 804-810.

[90] Kisely, S; Campbell, LA; Skerritt, P. Psychological interventions for symptomatic management of non-specific chest pain with normal coronary anatomy. Cochrane Database Syst Rev (Online), 2005, (1): Cochrane AN: CD004101.

[91] Tyni-Lenne, R; Stryjan, S; Eriksson, B;et al. Beneficial therapeutic effects of physical training and relaxation therapy in women with coronary syndrome X [J]. *Physiother. Res. Int.*, 2002, 7 (1): 35-43.

[92] Kronhaus, KD; Lawson, WE. Enhanced external counterpulsation is an effective treatment for Syndrome X [J]. *Int. J Cardiol.*, 2009 ,135 (2): 256-257.

[93] Zhang, MZ; Li, XM. Syndrome differentiation and treatment of traditional Chinese medicine on microvascular angina [J]. *The Journal of Practical Medicine*, 2001, 17(2): 177.

[94] Xu, LJ; Wang, WY. Effects of quickening the blood and transforming stasis method on blood endothelin-1 level and endothelium-dependent vasodilatated function in patients with syndrom X [J]. *Chinese Traditional Patent Medicine*, 2002, 24(7): 519-521.

[95] Lin, N. Treatment of 11 cases with syndrome X by *Qi* boosting and *Yang* warming method [J]. *Journal of Practical Traditional Chinese Internal Medicine*, 2007, 21(7): 68-69.

[96] Zhang, XY. Clinical experience of treatment for 48 patients with cardiac syndrome X by soothing Liver and regulating *Qi* [J]. *Journal of Emergency in Traditional Chinese Medicine*, 2008, 17(11): 1608-1609.

[97] Wu, HL; Hu, LN. Therapeutic observation on the method of regulating the spleen to protect the heart in treating myocardial microvascular Lesion [J]. *Henan Traditional Chinese Medicine*, 2009, 29(1): 45-46.

[98] Zhu, XH; Jia, YP. Clinical observation of decoction for removing blood stasis in the treatment of 30 cases of X-syndrome [J]. *Journal of Henan College of Traditional Chinese Medicine*, 2003, 2(3): 105.

[99] Zhang, XH; Song, QF. *Taohongsiwu* decoction for the treatment of 20 patients with syndrome X [J]. *Journal of Emergency in Traditional Chinese Medicine*, 2002, 2(4): 137.

[100]] Zhao, XD. Treatment of 38 patients with cardiac syndrome X by classic formulae [J]. *Henan Traditional Chinese Medicine*, 2003, 23(7): 10.

[101] Liu, H; Hu, YC. The effect of *Tongxinluo* on the vascular endothelial function in patients with syndrome X [J]. *Journal of Diffcult and Complicated Cases*, 2003, 4(8): 218.

[102] Bi, XP; Cai, XJ; Wei, F. Clinical effect observation of *Tongxinluo* capsule in treating patients with cardiac syndrome X [J]. *Hebei Medical Journal*, 2005, 27(8):587.

[103] Feng, ZB; Li, CM; Cheng, RN; et al. The Clinical Study of Cardiac X-syndrome Treated with *Tongxinluo* Capsule [J]. *Journal of Bethune Military Medical College*, 2005, 3(1): 25-26.

[104] Li, SY; Tang, Q. Clinical effect observation of *Tongxinluo* capsule combined with western medicine treatment in 36 Cases with cardiac syndrome X [J]. *Yunnan Journal of Traditional Chinese Medicine and Materia Medica*, 2009, 30(11): 15-16.

[105] Wang, LW; Wang. XB; Hu, YS; et al. Research on *Xuefuzhuyu* capsules for the treatment of cardiac syndrome X [J]. *Beijing Journal of Traditional Chinese Medicine*, 2003, 22(3): 65.

[106] Li, B; Mao, L; Chen, RY. Efficacy of Heart-protecting Musk Pill on patients with cardiac syndrome X [J] .*Chinese Journal of Integrative Medicine on Cardio-/Cerebrovascular Disease*, 2009, 7(1): 88-89.

[107] Niu, TF; Li, J; Qi, HX; et al. *XinXueAn* granular infusion for the treatment of 30 cases with cardiac syndrome X [J]. *Chinese Journal of Integrative Medicine on Cardio-/Cerebrovascular Disease*, 2008, 6(9): 1025-1026.

[108] Li JJ; Wang Y; Nie SP;et al. Xuezhikang, an extract of cholestin, decreases plasma inflammatory markers and endothelin-1, improve exercise-induced ischemia and subjective feelings in patients with cardiac syndrome X[J]. *Int. J. Cardiol*,2007,122 (1):82-4.

[109] Mao, JY; Zhang, ZP; Wang, HH; et al. Clinical analysis of 12 patients with Cardiac Syndrome X [J]. *Journal of Emergency in Traditional Chinese Medicine,* 2005, 14(4): 368-369.

[110] Mao, JY; Wang, HH; Ge, YB; et al. Analysis on the characteristics of TCM Syndrome in 51 patients with Cardiac Syndrome X [J]. *Journal of Traditional Chinese Medicine*, 2007, 48(12): 1111-1112.

[111] Mao, JY; Ge, YB; Wang, HH; et al. Summary of 32 Patients with Cardiac Syndrome X Treated by TCM Therapy Of Regulating *Qi* Relieving Chest Stuffiness and promoting Blood Circulation [J]. *Chinese Joumal of Integrative Medicine,* 2007, 13(l): 17-21.

[112] Wang, XL; Mao, JY; Wang, HH; et al. Clinical study on *Qi*-regulating, chest-relaxing and blood-activating therapy for Cardiac Syndrome X [J]. *Shanghai Journal of Traditional Chinese Medicine*, 2009, 43(1): 33-35.

[113] Johnson, BD; Shaw, LJ; Buchthal, SD; et al. Prognosis in women with myocardial ischemia in the absence of obstructive coronary disease: results from the National Institutes of Health-National. Heart, Lung, and Blood Institute-sponsored Women's Ischemia Syndrome Evaluation (WISE) [J]. *Circulation*, 2004, 109 (24): 2993-2999.

[114] Halcox, JP; Schenke, WH; Zalos, G; et al. Prognostic value of coronary vascular endothelial dysfunction [J]. *Circulation,* 2002, 106(6): 653-658.

In: Chest Pain Causes, Diagnosis and Treatment   ISBN 978-1-61728-112-9
Editor: Sophie M. Weber, pp. 35-64   © 2010 Nova Science Publishers, Inc.

Chapter 2

Scores for Likelihood Classification of Acute Coronary Syndrome: What is the Evidence?

Scott Goldberg,[1] Jonathan Ilgen [2] and Alex F. Manini[;11]
1. Department of Emergency Medicine, Mount Sinai School of Medicine,
New York, NY, USA
2. Department of Emergency Medicine, Oregon Heath and Science
University, Portland, OR, USA

Abstract

Despite decades of health outcomes research, a fail-safe way to rule out acute coronary syndrome (ACS) at the time of a patient's initial presentation remains elusive. Although there may be variability in the rates at which ACS is missed at individual hospitals, the "missed ACS rate" is generally inversely proportional to the rule-in rate. Predicting the patients who will ultimately be diagnosed with ACS is particularly problematic for that subset of patients with acute chest pain but with normal initial cardiac biomarkers and a non-diagnostic electrocardiogram.

[1] Corresponding Author: Dr. Manini can be reached by mail at Mt. Sinai School of Medicine, One Gustave L. Levy Drive, Box 1620, New York, NY 10029. Facsimile: 866-255-8229. Email: alex.manini@mountsinai.org.

This chapter will summarize the available prediction instruments that can be used for likelihood classification of ACS, including the most contemporary risk scores. How these tools address the need for intensive care and predict short-term prognosis will be explored. Data comparing these scores will also be reviewed. Lastly, a discussion of the pros, cons, and applications of several validated models to classify the presence or absence of ACS in undifferentiated ED populations will be presented.

Introduction

Scope

Acute coronary syndromes (ACS) include the spectrum of unstable angina pectoris (UAP), non-ST elevation myocardial infarction (NSTEMI), and ST-elevation myocardial infarction (STEMI) [60]. Upon the initial presentation to the emergency department (ED), it is essential for clinicians to identify patients with the highest likelihood of ACS, particularly NSTEMI, in order to guide diagnostic and therapeutic management based on published guidelines [2,63]. To improve resource use and ED efficiency, screening tools developed for use during the initial presentation must be diagnostically sensitive and accurate in order to assess the likelihood that the patient is presenting with ACS.

Patients presenting to the ED with chest pain or other symptoms consistent with ACS account for 5–8% of all ED visits [46]. Approximately 5-6 million people in the United States annually undergo evaluation in the ED for acute chest pain [1]. Of these, approximately 2-5% with acute myocardial infarction (AMI) are discharged inappropriately [56,65]. EDs using an unstructured, individualized approach to triage of patients with chest pain consume considerable health care resources for patients without coronary artery disease [17].

Likelihood Classification vs. Risk Stratification

Identifying patients with chest pain who have the highest likelihood of ACS is essential to the initial ED diagnostic and therapeutic management plan [13,15]. However, patients with negative cardiac biomarkers and a non-diagnostic ECG may still be at risk for adverse events in the short term and beyond. As such, risk stratification is the process of identifying patients who are at highest risk of future adverse events following a presentation with a suspected ACS [63].

On the initial presentation of a patient with acute chest pain, the physician first must determine the likelihood that the presenting symptoms are consistent with possible ACS; this is likelihood classification. Likelihood classification is usually conducted by emergency physicians, admitting physicians, or clinicians referring patients from clinics for expedited hospital evaluation. The process of likelihood classification for ACS typically takes into account elements of the history and physical examination, the patient's prior medical history—which may or may not be immediately available to the clinician at the time of presentation—and a limited set of diagnostic tests that include an ECG and cardiac biomarkers.

Risk stratification, on the other hand, refers to a patient's risk of a particular outcome (e.g., mortality) over time. This is often performed at the time of admission to a chest pain unit or inpatient unit by the admitting physicians. Risk assessment tools may then be applied to guide the clinician regarding the patient's prognosis, need for additional testing, and other therapeutic options.

Outcomes in the Chest Pain Score Literature

A major limitation of chest pain score research is that unlike for AMI [38], there is no established gold standard to define UAP. Thus, studies commonly incorporate use of an adjudication panel of experts to define ACS (i.e., the combination of UAP, NSTEMI, and STEMI). Commonly, studies may also utilize a composite endpoint which usually includes the combination of death, AMI, and revascularization (typically defined as at least one of either percutaneous coronary intervention or coronary artery bypass grafting).

Additionally, timing of detection of outcomes varies across different studies and varies anywhere from 72 hours, to 30 days, or even as far out as one year. For the above reasons, standardized reporting guidelines for chest pain research studies have been created and endorsed by such organizations as the American College of Emergency Physicians, American Heart Association, American College of Cardiology, and the Society for Academic Emergency Medicine [38].

To confound the issue of outcomes further, many studies evaluating the diagnostic approach to undifferentiated acute chest pain have additional limitations, such as the common exclusion of patients with STEMI, as this cohort has a clearly developed, expedited management approach [47]. Further complicating a critical appraisal of the literature, the definition of ACS has evolved during the decades when several chest pain risk scores were developed [60]. Thus, when applying a particular risk score to a patient with undifferentiated acute chest pain, one must be mindful of the outcome(s) that the tool was designed to predict when derived and validated.

Objectives of this Chapter

The aim of this chapter is to provide an assessment of the literature regarding scores for likelihood classification of suspected ACS. Although a normal ECG and negative cardiac biomarkers at presentation predicts a relatively lower risk for complications, it cannot absolutely exclude UAP or AMI [10,32,66,76]. Furthermore, classic cardiac risk factors have little role in predicting the cause of acute chest pain [66]. Therefore in order to be useful to clinicians, a clinical tool that predicts the likelihood of ACS needs to outperform the modest predictive capacity that the initial ECG, cardiac biomarkers, and traditional cardiac risk factors have in isolation. Principles of risk score use for post-myocardial infarction risk stratification (such as GUSTO [11], PREDICT [42], InTimeII [58], Braunwald classification [12], and PURSUIT [7]) and issues regarding the utility/safety/cost-effectiveness of chest pain unit (CPU) protocols and stress testing protocols are beyond the scope of this chapter and have been covered in detail elsewhere [19,27,49,63,75].

Scores for Classification of Acute Chest Pain

As discussed above, up to 5% of patients with symptoms suggestive of ACS are inappropriately discharged from the ED [56,65]. Patients with AMI who are mistakenly discharged from the ED have short-term mortality rates of about 25 percent, at least twice what would be expected if they were admitted [50]. A clinician's initial diagnostic impression of "noncardiac" chest pain is notoriously unreliable [57]. Risk prediction instruments or "scores" attempt to improve clinicians' diagnostic accuracy and aid prognosis by incorporating information (demographic, historical, physical examination, ECG, and other findings) that is readily available at the bedside to produce an objective assessment of likelihood classification or risk stratification.

Using scores to aid clinical decision making is not without peril, and many caveats and limitations must be considered prior to incorporation into one's practice. For example, many authors draw attention to the potential flaws of chest pain risk scores derived from datasets of clinical trials. These databases typically include a highly-selected patient population, many with a high pretest probability of ACS (or even already-established AMI). Moreover, some risk scores require data that is not readily available or cumbersome to collect in the ED, while others predate emerging technologies (e.g., new generation highly-sensitive cardiac biomarkers). These scores thus may not accurately represent the realities of current clinical practice. Accordingly, a clinician must put these studies into context and be careful about generalizing the results to one's own patient population. Examples of the most significant score limitations include any of the following: (a) requirement for detailed information which may not be readily available during the initial stabilization (e.g., Killip class, imaging results from outside institutions); (b) highly-selected patient enrollment (i.e., poor generalizability); (c) exclusion of new or emerging prognostic variables; and (d) research design applicable to either patients with NSTEMI or STEMI, but not both (i.e., more generalizability issues). These issues are clarified during the discussion of each relevant risk assessment tool below.

History, Physical Examination, and Initial Electrocardiogram

While advancements in ancillary testing have made vast improvements in recent years, the cornerstone of clinical diagnosis of ACS still lies in the history and physical examination. Most studies evaluating historical and physical findings and their relation to ischemic chest pain compare patients *with* AMI to those *without* AMI, neglecting the challenge of diagnosing UAP and thus limiting the generalizability of these studies to the full spectrum of ACS. However, it is useful to note the particular pattern of historical and physical findings associated with established AMI.

Two recent reviews [61,77] have explored the physical findings that impact the likelihood a patient's symptoms represent an acute AMI. Among the descriptors of chest pain, *sharp* or *stabbing* have the strongest likelihood ratios (LR) negative for AMI (LR 0.3), while *pressure* correlates very little or not at all (LR 1.3) [77]. Pain radiating to the right (LR 2.9-4.7) or both arms (LR 4.1-7.1) increases the likelihood of AMI more than radiation to the left arm (LR 2.0-2.3), yet there was no association between the severity of pain and AMI [61,77]. Pain that is positional (LR 0.3), pleuritic (LR 0.2), or reproducible with palpation (LR 0.3) all decrease the likelihood of AMI [77]. While association of pain with exertion modestly increases likelihood of AMI (LR 2.3), relief with nitroglycerin does not [36]. The associated symptoms of nausea or vomiting (LR 1.9) and diaphoresis (LR 2.0) both increase likelihood of AMI [77]. Most importantly, however, no single element of the chest pain history conveys a powerful enough LR to safely discharge a patient without additional testing. The impact of various historical features and examination findings on the likelihood of ACS is summarized in **Table 1**. Additionally, Panju and colleagues examined the utility of ECG to support the diagnosis of AMI, and these findings are summarized in **Table 2**.

Tierney et al. [78] attempted to combine findings from the history, physical examination, and initial ECG into a risk prediction model. They used features of the history (prior MI), physical examination (diaphoresis with chest pain), and ECG (any ST elevation and new pathological Q waves) coupled with initial serum cardiac biomarkers. When compared to unstructured physician assessment, this four-point risk score was slightly less sensitive for AMI (80.6% v 87.1%, p=NS) but showed improved specificity (86.0% v 78.5%, p<0.01) and accuracy (85.4% v 79.4%, p<0.05).

Table 1. History And Physical Findings Associated With Likelihood Of AMI

	Symptoms	Likelihood Ratio (95% CI)	
		Swap [78]	Panju [61]
Increased Likelihood	Radiation to right arm\shoulder	4.7 (1.9-1.2)	2.9 (1.4-6.0)
	Radiation to both arms or shoulders	4.1 (2.5-6.5)	7.1 (3.6-14.2)
	Association with exertion	2.4 (1.5-3.8)	
	Radiation to left arm	2.3 (1.7-3.1)	2.3 (1.7-3.1)
	Diaphoresis	2.0 (1.9-2.2)	2.0 (1.9-2.2)
	Nausea or vomiting	1.9 (1.7-2.3)	1.9 (1.7-2.3)
	Pain worse than previous angina or similar to previous MI	1.8 (1.6-2.0)	-
	Pressure	1.3 (1.2-1.5)	-
	Third heart sound	-	3.2 (1.6-6.5)
	Pulmonary crackles	-	2.1 (1.4-3.1)
Decreased Likelihood	Pleuritic	0.2 (0.1-0.3)	0.2 (0.2-0.3)
	Positional	0.3 (0.2-0.5)	0.3 (0.2-0.4)
	Sharp	0.3 (0.2-0.5)	0.3 (0.2-0.5)
	Reproducible with palpation	0.3 (0.2-0.4)	0.3 (0.2-0.4)
	Inframammary	0.8 (0.7-0.9)	-
	Not associated with exertion	0.8 (0.6-0.9)	-

Abbreviations: AMI = acute myocardial infarction; CI = confidence interval; MI = myocardial infarction.

Table 2. ECG Findings Associated With Myocardial Infarction

ECG Finding	Likelihood Ratio (95% CI)[*]	
New ST elevation ≥ 1mm	5.9-53.9	
New Q wave	5.3-24.8	
Any ST elevation	11.2	(7.1-17.8)
New conduction defect	6.3	(2.5-15.7)
New ST depression	3.0-5.2	
Any Q wave	3.9	(2.7-5.7)
Any ST depression	3.2	(2.5-4.1)
T wave peaking or inversion ≥ 1mm	3.1	
New T wave inversion	2.4-2.8	
Any conduction defect	2.7	(1.4-5.4)
Normal ECG	0.1-0.3	

* Likelihood ratios are reported in ranges in heterogeneous studies and with confidence intervals if available.

Abbreviations: CI = confidence intervals; ECG = electrocardiogram; mm = millimeter.

Traditional Cardiac Risk Factors: Framingham

The identification of risk factors for the development of coronary heart disease provided a powerful link between the fields of cardiology and preventive medicine [22]. In practice, the very same traditional cardiac risk factors derived from the population followed in the classic Framingham Study (gender, age, hypertension, diabetes mellitus, tobacco smoking, hyperlipidemia, family history, menopause, and cocaine use) are routinely gathered by clinicians for use in the assessment of individual patients with acute chest pain [33].

More recently, the Framingham Risk Score was developed as a percentage from 0-100. It is calculated by incorporating demographics (age, sex), past medical history (diabetes, smoking), blood pressure measurement, and serum cholesterol levels [83]. Based on consensus guidelines, scores are categorized as low (0-9%), intermediate (10-20%), and high (>20%) based on recommendations from the Second Joint Task Force of European and other Societies on Coronary Prevention [84]. However, this score was validated to assess the 10-year risk of development of coronary heart disease and is not recommended for use in the likelihood estimation of ACS in acute chest pain.

What about the utility of relying upon cardiac risk factor burden on the ED diagnosis of ACS? Han and colleagues [35] recently studied the impact of traditional cardiac risk factor burden in the ED population with acute chest pain. The results were clear—there was limited added value in diagnosing ACS, especially for patients over 40 years old. To explain these results, it is important to remember that Bayesian analysis indicates that risk factors are a population phenomenon rather than the likelihood of a condition in any individual patient. Thus, the presence of a population risk factor, or a collection of risk factors, is far less important in diagnosing ACS in the ED than the individual's history of presenting illness, the presence of ST segment or T wave changes, or cardiac biomarker abnormalities. Thus, while clinicians regularly gather information on Framingham risk factors to clinically assess likelihood of ACS in the acute ED setting, the role should actually be minimized.

Goldman Score

Goldman and colleagues derived some of the earliest diagnostic algorithms for patients with acute chest pain [31-32]. These decision aids address two important issues frequently encountered in the ED: identifying individuals with true myocardial AMI or UAP within a cohort of patients with undifferentiated chest pain, and estimating the short-term risk of major cardiac complications in this group of patients as a means to influence admission decisions.

Goldman et al. published their first cardiac risk stratification algorithm in 1982 [34]. This study devised an algorithm to improve the specificity for predicting AMI among patients *admitted* with chest pain. Patients were eligible for enrollment if they were over 25 years of age (30 years in derivation set) and had an acute complaint of anterior, precordial, or left-lateral chest pain. No other ischemic symptoms were included for enrollment purposes. To derive the algorithm, investigators collected extensive relevant data (historical and demographic information, medication usage, physical examination and EKG findings, in-hospital and outpatient course) on 482 patients evaluated by trainees at one tertiary care hospital. To derive the algorithm, recursive partitioning was employed to retrospectively derive a decision tree (see **Figure 1**) that identified 100% of patients with AMI. To test the algorithm, it was prospectively applied at another hospital in a similar ED patient population with good results: 91% sensitivity for AMI, 70% specificity for non-infarction, and overall accuracy of 73%. When compared to physicians' unstructured decision to admit patients to the CCU, the model improved physicians' specificity for non-infarction (77% vs. 67%) and overall accuracy for AMI (79% vs. 71%), while sensitivity remained similar (88% vs. 91%). At the algorithm's terminal endpoints patients could be subdivided into risk groups with 72-hour rates of AMI as low as 1-4%.

A similar derivation and validation scheme was published by the same authors in 1988, with the new aim of identifying patients at risk for major cardiac complications [31]. A protocol was derived using recursive portioning on data collected from 1379 patients with chest pain. This new protocol, with sequential branch points concerning historical, demographic, and electrocardiographic changes, was prospectively validated in 4770 patients at two university and four community hospitals.

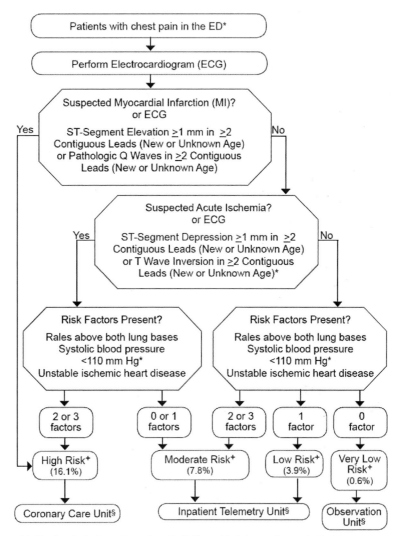

* Modifications in decision rule employed by Reilly et al. include: enrollment of only patients admitted with diagnosis of suspected acute cardiac ischemic, left bundle branch block (new or unknown age) as a criteria for acute ischemia and systolic blood pressure <100 mm Hg rather than <110 as a risk factor.
+ Percentages reflect rate of major cardiac complications durıng validation phase by Goldman et al. (1996).
§ Suggested triage based on clinical decision rule by Reilly et al.

Figure 1. The Goldman algorithm for triage of patients with acute chest pain in the emergency department.

The investigators measured the rate of emergent complications requiring intensive care, including tachydysrhythmia, need for cardioversion or pacemaker placement, cardiogenic shock, or cardiac or respiratory arrest. Compared to unstructured physician decisions, the protocol had significantly higher specificity (74% vs. 71%) and overall accuracy (76% vs. 73%) for AMI, though sensitivity was unchanged (88% vs. 87.8%). In a similar fashion to the decision tree described in 1982, however, subgroups deemed to be "non-MI" based on this algorithm had AMI rates of 1-8% during prospective validation. The rate of complications within 72-hours of presentation were highest in patients with AMI (16%), and rates of these events were highest when the physicians and the protocol concurred with the decision to admit the patient to the CCU (7.5%), similar when the physician and computer disagreed (1.5%), and low when neither recommended admission (0.35%).

Dubbed as the "Goldman score" or "Goldman algorithm" the same authors studied the presenting clinical features in patients with chest pain that predicted major cardiac events within 72 hours [32]. Derived from a population of 10,682 patients at three university and four community hospitals, this algorithm defined a spectrum of risk across four subgroups of patients based on clinical data available at the time of ED evaluation. This decision tree was prospectively employed on 4,676 patients at an urban tertiary care hospital. The algorithm and rates of major events are shown in Figure 1. Of note, the authors caution that "after an initial period of 12 hours, the development of an event was more important than the patient's original risk factors in predicting the probability of a subsequent event."

With minor modifications, the Goldman score was studied at an urban county hospital to assess impact on physician disposition decisions for patients with chest pain, concurrently studying whether patient outcomes were affected [68]. Patients were enrolled only if they were admitted with a suspected diagnosis of ACS (both with and without chest pain), though a separate cohort was enrolled consisting of patients who were discharged directly from the ED in order to minimize recruitment bias. Upon enrollment, patients were triaged to inpatient beds based on their Goldman risk group (see Figure 1), and patients were tracked for 72 hours. The primary outcomes measured were safety and efficiency. "Safety" represented the proportion of all patients who subsequently experienced major cardiac complications within 72 hours, indicating appropriate triage to the coronary care or telemetry unit upon admission. "Efficiency" was defined as the proportion of patients who did not experience these complications who had been initially admitted to an unmonitored ward or the ED observation unit. Among 1008 with complete data upon enrollment, there was a 3.5% major cardiac complication rate. There were no complications among the cohort discharged directly from the ED. When compared to the pre-intervention group, the Goldman protocol improved "efficiency" (36 vs. 21%), with no change in "safety" (94% vs. 89%), indicating the modest utility of this risk score for appropriate triage of ED patients with suspected ACS.

Limkakeng et al., used the Goldman score in conjunction with a negative troponin I (cTnI) assay to assess whether these, in combination, could identify a population of patients at ED presentation that would be safe for discharge [51]. Safety was defined as patients at <1% risk for death, AMI, and revascularization within 30 days. Using a Goldman 72-hour risk of $\leq$ 4% and cTnI threshold of $\leq$ 0.3 ng/ml, these investigators failed to find a low risk population among the 998 patients who met enrollment criteria. Despite the combination of low clinical risk based on this algorithm and a negative initial cTnI, 4.9% of patients met the composite endpoint of major cardiac event and 2.3% had an AMI. More recently, Manini and colleagues [54] evaluated the Goldman score in ED patients who met criteria for the Ruling out Myocardial Infarction using Cardiac Computed Angiography Tomography study (ROMICAT) [37] and found that even in the lowest Goldman risk group 30-day ACS rates were unacceptably high. Based on the above two studies, it appears that using the Goldman Score to identify a subpopulation of ED patients amenable for safe discharge is flawed.

Acute Cardiac Ischemia Time Insensitive Predictive Instrument (ACI-TIPI)

Selker and colleagues originally developed the Acute Cardiac Ischemia Time-Insensitive Predictive Instrument (ACI-TIPI) as a risk stratification tool for use by clinicians in real-time [72]. The ACI-TIPI computes a 0-100 percent probability that a given patient has ACS. It is based on a logistic regression equation that uses demographics (age and gender), presenting symptoms (chest pain as chief complaint or not), and ECG variables (ST segment deviation, Q waves, and T-wave abnormalities), and is applicable to any ED patient presenting with any symptom suggestive of ACS. Originally in a handheld calculator form, it is now incorporated into conventional electrocardiographs so that the patient's ACI-TIPI probability is printed with the standard ECG header text. In the initial derivation, the use of the ACI-TIPI model was associated with reduced hospitalization among ED patients without acute cardiac ischemia, while appropriate admission for UAP or AMI was not affected [73].

Studies investigating the use of ACI-TIPI as a surrogate of pretest probability for outcomes of cardiac stress test results have yielded mixed results. The ability of ACI-TIPI to predict exercise treadmill test results in "low-risk" patients was studied by Manini and colleagues [53]. Patients were enrolled if they had negative initial cardiac biomarkers, an initial ECG without new or ischemic changes, and clinical judgment by the attending physician that the patient was at low risk of a poor outcome. They found that ACI-TIPI of ≥20% independently predicted non-negative treadmill test outcomes when controlled for potential confounding variables. A study by Welch and colleagues [82] evaluated performance of ACI-TIPI, compared to raw physician assessment, in patients who received myocardial perfusion imaging with 99mTc sestamibi. The study found no improvement in pretest probability with ACI-TIPI, and the authors concluded that ACI-TIPI did not permit for more selective imaging with rest sestamibi to aid the triage of low to moderate risk patients with suspected ACS.

Two systematic reviews of available cardiac risk stratification technologies by the National Heart Attack Alert Program have graded the evidence supporting ACI-TIPI as Class A ("least bias"), one of only three tools along with the Goldman score and artificial neural networks (both discussed in separate sections of this chapter) to receive this rating [48,74]. Clinical use of ACI-TIPI, however, must be tempered with the major limitation that the instrument overestimates the true incidence of disease in the lower probability ranges [72].

Thrombolysis in Myocardial Infarction (TIMI) Score

Antman and colleagues [3] derived a clinical prediction rule for risk assessment of patients with UAP and NSTEMI from the cohort of patients in the Thrombolytics In Myocardial Infarction (TIMI) 11b study [4,71] (see Table 3).

Table 3. Thrombolysis In Myocardial Infarction (TIMI) Risk Score (Max. Score = 7)

Factor:	Points Assigned:
Age ≥ 65 Years	1
≥ 3 CAD Risk Factors	1
Use of ASA in Past 7 Days	1
Known CAD with Stenosis ≥ 50%	1
> 1 Episode of Angina at Rest in Past 24h	1
ST-segment Deviation	1
Elevated Cardiac Biomarkers	1

Abbreviations: ASA = aspirin; CAD = coronary artery disease; h = hour; max = maximum.

At that time, the available validated prediction rules (e.g., Goldman, Framingham) did not necessarily provide accurate prognostic information given novel therapies for [2,47], and redefinitions of [60], ACS. After an early attempt at a simple risk-stratification tool [41], this group derived a seven point score dubbed the TIMI Risk Score (TRS) from a population of patients with confirmed ACS. The authors argued that the TRS contained several advantages over previous risk score models particularly that it consisted of a small number of discrete, dichotomous variables, readily available at the bedside or in real-time evaluation of patients. However, it was derived from a cohort of patients with known ACS, potentially limiting its generalizability to an undifferentiated chest pain population [3,14,59].

After its initial derivation, the TRS was applied to both the TIMI-11b and ESSENCE cohorts, showing an incremental increase in the risk of all-cause mortality within 14 days with rising scores [4]. Further, the benefit of enoxaparin rose in conjunction with rising risk scores, indicating the TRS could be employed for therapeutic decision-making as well [3]. The TRS was subsequently validated in several large cohorts. The TACTICS-TIMI trial [14] demonstrated an increased rate of death, MI or ACS within 6 months with an increased TRS. It further showed an incremental benefit of an early invasive strategy in those receiving tirofiban, a glycoprotein 2a/3b inhibitor, with increasing TRS. The PRISM-PLUS trial [59] demonstrated an increasing risk of death, MI or urgent revascularization within 14 days with increasing TRS, as well as an incremental increase in the benefit of tirofiban with increasing TRS. These studies suggested the applicability of the TRS to a wider spectrum of patient populations, with varied end points and duration of prognostic value

(6 months versus the 14 days in the initial derivation). Since then the TRS has been shown to provide prognostic information up to 1 year [71,81]. While the prognostic value of the TRS has been validated within a well-defined population with confirmed ACS, it was not initially studied in a cohort of patients with undifferentiated chest pain. Given its simplicity and easy application at the bedside, however, the TRS was an attractive candidate for applicability in the ED which led to further study of a more generalizable patient population. Initial work exploring the application of TRS to an ED population found that many more patients had low TRSs than those in the initial derivation (which had had a normal distribution of scores) [3,16,64].

Subpopulations with chest pain were also studied including cocaine users [64] and STEMI patients [16], populations previously excluded from trials utilizing the TRS yet prevalent in the ED setting. Both cohorts found that rising TRS were associated with a higher rate of major cardiac complications. However, a TRS of 0 still carried an approximately 2% chance of adverse outcomes in both trials, failing to achieve a lower rate of missed ACS than the baseline rate of inappropriate discharge for patients with AMI discussed above [20,56,65]. Even patients with a TRS of 0 and a clinical impression of an "alternative diagnosis" still carried an adverse event rate up to 3% [13].

Subsequent work has shown that patients with both a low TRS (score 0-2) and a low clinical suspicion of ACS, who then undergo a negative coronary CT, have a <1% 30 day adverse outcome rate [39]. It should be noted that a subsequent trial of an undifferentiated ED chest pain population with recent cocaine use failed to demonstrate the same utility of the TRS [15]. In addition, females may have different 30-day outcome profiles (death, MI, revascularization) at similar TRS than males, calling into question its prognostic utility in women [45].

Several modifications of TRS have been made in attempts to improve diagnostic and prognostic performance. Multiple studies have found the serum troponin concentration to be the single strongest prognostic indicator among all components of the TRS [16,43,64,79]. Conway and colleagues [18] demonstrated that by excluding troponin from the TRS, the "front door" score still had prognostic value but suffered from a decreased sensitivity and specificity. When the TRS is modified to include heart failure and diabetes [28] or to include only the strongest prognostic indicators (age, existing coronary stenosis, elevated troponin, and ST segment changes on presenting ECG) [43], these changes trade increased prognostic value at the price of decreased sensitivity. Recently, Manini and colleagues [54] performed a secondary analysis on a cohort who underwent cardiac CT angiography to assess the diagnostic test characteristics of TRS for ACS within 30-days. TRS performed poorly (less than 58% sensitivity and 91% specificity), again highlighting the limited utility of the TRS to estimate likelihood of ACS in undifferentiated chest pain [54].

In summary, while the TRS provides valuable prognostic information to guide medical therapy, it does not perform well to safely exclude ACS even in the lowest risk category. A score of 0 is still associated with adverse event rates of 1-6% in various studies [3,14,16,43,64]. Thus, while the TRS functions best when used to risk stratify prognosis of adverse events, especially in a high risk ACS population [3,69], it has limited utility for likelihood classification of ACS in an undifferentiated ED chest pain population.

Global Registry of Acute Coronary Events (GRACE) and Platelet Glycoprotein IIb/IIIa in Unstable Angina: Receptor Suppression Using Integrilin Trial (PURSUIT)

The GRACE [26] and PURSUIT [7] scores were derived essentially to explore the effect of additional risk factors on the prognostic accuracy of TRS. Like the TRS, both of these risk scores were derived from subjects with confirmed ACS. In the derivation cohorts, GRACE and PURSUIT both had better discriminatory accuracy for adverse cardiac events than the TRS at 1 year follow-up [23,86]. When compared individually, all three scores were better than unstructured physician risk assessment at predicting long-term patient outcomes [86]. Importantly, when employed in a population with undifferentiated chest pain, the GRACE score and the TRS performed equally well in predicting 30 day outcomes though GRACE was marginally better at predicting 3 month composite outcomes [52,67]. In clinical practice, the real-time calculation of the GRACE score requires large amounts of data collection and use of a calculator. For these reasons, GRACE has not gained widespread acceptance among clinicians for initial likelihood classification of ACS [23,85].

Sanchis/Geleijnse Score

A novel risk model was recently established by Sanchis and colleagues to predict mortality or AMI at one-year in low risk patients with chest pain [70]. The Sanchis score is based on 18 criteria derived from the work of Geleijnse and colleagues [29], as well as 4 additional historical elements. The score ranges from 0-6 based on the following scoring system: Geleijnse chest pain score at least 10 (1 point), 2 or more chest pain episodes within 24 hours (1 point), age greater than 66 years (1 point), insulin dependent diabetes mellitus (2 points), and prior percutaneous transluminal coronary angioplasty (1 point). Risk categories are assigned according to score: low-risk (0-1 points), intermediate-risk (2 points), and high-risk (3-6 points). This point system classifies patients into five progressive risk categories, with 1-year death and AMI rates from 0% to 29% depending on risk category—and more accurately predicts death rate and AMI at one year than the TRS [70].

Manini and colleagues [54] evaluated the diagnostic performance of the Sanchis score for 30-day ACS on a cohort who underwent cardiac CT angiography. Predictably, even the lowest risk group had poor sensitivity and did not identify a group amenable for safe discharge without further testing. Given these results, combined with the impracticality of collecting and sorting 25 clinical variables in a busy ED setting, the Sanchis score has gained limited acceptance by clinicians.

Artificial Neural Networks

Artificial neural networks are computer algorithms that use several data inputs to estimate, using non-linear equations, the probability of a specific outcome or output as a mathematical correlate to the clinical practice of pattern recognition. Neural networks attempt to classify patients' likelihood of AMI, based on risk factors derived from a registry of ED patients. As will be discussed, these studies found that artificial neural networks could achieve a high sensitivity and high specificity for AMI, but had little impact on actual clinical decision-making.

Baxt and colleagues prospectively derived the diagnostic performance of an artificial neural network on physician-completed questionnaires of 331 patients presenting with anterior chest pain [5]. The blinded investigators collected elements of the patients' medical history, physical findings, and ECG results to produce a multivariate prediction model for diagnosis of AMI based on CK/CK-MB, LDH isoenzyme-1, ECG findings, or sestamibi imaging results (**Table 4**). This same artificial neural network was prospectively validated in a population of 1,070 patients at a major, urban teaching hospital with only 3% of subjects lost to follow-up [6].

In a real-time external validation study, however, the neural network was unable to improve the admission decision for ED patients with chest pain [40]. Authors have pointed to other limitations of neural networks such as the exclusion of UAP in the original studies as well as difficulties of incorporating non-linear statistical models into a busy clinical practice. For these reasons, there is poor widespread acceptance of artificial neural networks for likelihood classification of ACS.

Table 4. Variables coded in artificial neural networks to predict AMI

Current History	Previous History	Examination	ECG
Age, Gender	Angina	JVD	2mm ST elevation
Left anterior location	Diabetes	Rates	1mm ST elevation
Radiation of pain	Hypertension		ST depression
Nausea and vomiting	Prior MI		T wave inversion
Faintness			Ischemic change
Sweating			
SOB			
Palpitations			
Response to NTG			

Abbreviations: AMI = acute myocardial infarction; ECG = electrocardiogram; MI = myocardial infarction; SOB = shortness of breath; NTG = nitroglycerin;

Risk Scores in Subpopulations

Given the limited utility of risk scores to identify very low risk patients who can be safely discharged without prolonged observation or inpatient admission, myriad approaches have been made in subpopulations, particularly women and young adults. Importantly, these scores should not be adopted into clinical practice until sufficient validation has occurred. Below, selected promising risk scores are discussed.

Risk Scores for Women

In chest pain literature from the late 1990's, women with confirmed AMI were reported to more likely present with "atypical" chest pain features [9,30,62]. Douglas and Ginsburg initially created a scoring system incorporating classic cardiac risk factors into determinants of risk using a literature review, with only modest clinical applicability due to high event rates (~20%) in the "low risk" group [25].

Subsequently, in 2004 Diercks and colleagues set out to define and validate a more definitive risk prediction instrument for ACS that is to be used specifically for women [24]. The authors retrospectively enrolled women with suspected ACS, negative initial cardiac biomarkers, and non-diagnostic ECG at presentation, then evaluated 30-day composite outcome (AMI, positive provocative study, or death). In a unicenter derivation group of 1,000 women, risk factors for the composite outcome included history of CAD, age >60 and "high suspicion" of ACS. In a unicenter validation set of over 2,500 women, this predictive instrument performed with modest sensitivity and specificity (76% and 78%, respectively), though these test characteristics outperformed both Goldman and ACI-TIPI scores (both discussed above). Unfortunately, poor inter-rater reliability, high rate of patients lost to follow-up (~20%), and lack of prospective external validation limits widespread adoption of this risk score.

Vancouver Chest Pain Rule

The Vancouver Chest Pain Rule [20] utilizes criteria that include age <40, low risk pain characteristics (non-radiating, pleuritic nature, and reproducibility), and a repeat set of cardiac biomarkers at 2 hr to determine eligibility for safe early discharge home. In a small prospective derivation cohort, the rule performed with >95% sensitivity for detection of the 30-day ACS. While promising, the lack of a clear gold standard for ACS may hinder its widespread adoption pending replication and validation.

Rule for Young Adults

In 2005, Marsan and colleagues [55] published their prospective validation of a rule derived in 2001 [80] from a cohort of patients aged 24-39. The rule incorporates classic cardiac risk factors, prior cardiac history and a non-diagnostic ECG to predict a composite outcome (death, AMI, revascularization) at 30 days. In the validation set of over 1,000 patients, a group with <2% composite outcome rate was identified. The rule is further improved by incorporating the results of the first set of cardiac biomarkers. While promising, this risk score suffers from a variety of methodological concerns which limits its clinical application until replication and further external validation is obtained.

Consensus Guidelines (AHA, AHCPR, AND AHRQ)

The American Heart Association (AHA) has published separate clinical practice guidelines for the approach to UAP/NSTEMI [2] and STEMI [47]. With regard to early risk stratification, a Class IC recommendation (procedure is useful/effective based on only expert opinion, case series, or standard-of-care) is made for "rapid clinical determination of the likelihood risk (i.e., high, intermediate, low) of obstructive CAD" in all patients with chest discomfort or symptoms suggestive of ACS. To determine the "likelihood risk," the authors suggest using high risk features (such as "accelerating tempo of symptoms" and pulmonary edema) adapted from another executive panel published by the Agency for Health Care Policy and Research (AHCPR) in 1994 [8]. However, the 1994 guidelines are now published with the following disclaimer: "THIS DOCUMENT IS NO LONGER VIEWED AS GUIDANCE FOR CURRENT MEDICAL PRACTICE."

With regard to risk scores for use in the initial approach to acute chest pain, the AHA guidelines for UAP/NSTEMI [2] state the following: "Use of risk-stratification models, such as the Thrombolysis In Myocardial Infarction (TIMI) or Global Registry of Acute Coronary Events (GRACE) risk score or the Platelet Glycoprotein IIb/IIIa in Unstable Angina: Receptor Suppression Using Integrilin Therapy (PURSUIT) risk model, can be useful to assist in decision making with regard to treatment options in patients with suspected ACS." This is issued as a Class IIB recommendation (in favor of procedure being useful/effective based on conflicting evidence from nonrandomized studies), but note that the scores are recommended only with regard to planning "treatment options." Unfortunately, no definitive AHA recommendations are made with regard to use of risk scores for the purpose of likelihood classification of ACS.

In 2001, the Agency for Healthcare Research and Quality (AHRQ) published a rigorous review of the literature evaluating technologies to diagnose ACS in the ED [49]. In the summary recommendations, the authors concluded that among all risk scoring technologies available at the time, "ACI-TIPI was shown to have the best triage accuracy for patients with acute cardiac ischemia and to be the most cost-effective technology." However, the authors emphasized that some technologies remain under-evaluated, the number of studies on the clinical impact of these technologies inadequate, and the quality of reporting by studies in this area need to be improved.

Conclusion

Evaluation of acute chest pain remains a clinical challenge despite the advent of several tools to evaluate risk for subsequent adverse cardiovascular events. While a diverse array of technologies exist to aid diagnosis of ACS at the time of initial presentation, there is no single scoring instrument that can identify all ACS patients and at the same time avoid hospitalizing many patients without ACS. Though a normal ECG at presentation predicts a lower risk for complications, it too cannot absolutely exclude ACS. Furthermore, classic cardiac risk factors have little role in the likelihood classification of an individual patient. In summary, while many risk scores have been rigorously studied, no currently validated risk scores may be used to effectively exclude ACS at the time of a patient's initial presentation. There is an urgent need for the development of highly sensitive and accurate risk assessment tools for acute chest pain in order to improve resource use and ED efficiency.

References

[1]   American Heart Association (1998). Heart and Stroke 1998 Statistical Update. Chicago, IL: *American Heart Association.*

[2]   Anderson, J.L., Adams, C.D., Antman, E.M., et al. (2007). ACC/AHA 2007 guidelines for the management of patients with unstable angina/non-ST-elevation myocardial infarction: executive summary. *Circulation*, 116, 803–877.

[3]   Antman, E.M., Cohen, M., Bernink, P.J., et al. (2000). The TIMI risk score for unstable angina/non-ST elevation MI: A method for prognostication and therapeutic decision making. *JAM*, 284, 835-42.

[4]   Antman, E.M., McCabe, C.H., Gurfinkel, E.P., et al. (1999). Enoxaparin prevents death and cardiac ischemic events in unstable angina/non-Q-wave myocardial infarction: results of the Thrombolysis in Myocardial Infarction (TIMI) 11B trial. *Circulation*, 100, 1593-1601.

[5]   Baxt, W.G. (1991). Use of an artificial neural network for the diagnosis of myocardial infarction. Ann Intern Med, 115, 843-8. Erratum in: Ann Intern Med 1992 Jan 1;116(1):94.

[6]   Baxt, W.G. and Skora, J. (1996). Prospective validation of artificial neural network trained to identify acute myocardial infarction. *Lancet*, 347, 12-5.

[7]   Boersma, E., Pieper, K.S., Steyerberg, E.W., et al. (2000). Predictors of outcome in patients with acute coronary syndromes without persistent ST-segment elevation: Results from an international trial of 9461 patients. The PURSUIT Investigators. *Circulation*, 101, 2557-67.

[8]   Braunwald, E., Mark, D.B., Jones, R.H., et al. (1994). Unstable Angina: Diagnosis and Management. Clinical Practice Guideline Number 10. AHCPR Publication No. 94-0602. Rockville, MD: Agency for Health Care Policy and Research and the National Heart, Lung, and Blood Institute, Public Health Service, U.S. Department of Health and Human Services. May 1994 (amended).

[9]   Brscic, E., Brusca, A., Presbitero, et al. (1997). Ischemic chest pain and global T-wave inversion in women with normal coronary angiograms. *Am. J. Cardiol.*, 80, 245–7.

[10] Brush, J.E. Jr., Brand, D.A., Acampora, D., et al. (1985). Use of the initial electrocardiogram to predict in-hospital complications of acute myocardial infarction. *N. Engl. J. Med.*, 312, 1137-41.

[11] Califf, R.M., Pieper, K.S., Lee, K.L., et al. (2000). Prediction of 1-year survival after thrombolysis for acute myocardial infarction in the global utilization of streptokinase and TPA for occluded coronary arteries trial. *Circulation*, 101, 2231–2238.

[12] Calvin, J.E., Klein, L.W., VandenBerg, B.J., et al. (1995). Risk stratification in unstable angina: prospective validation of the Braunwald classification. *JAMA*, 273, 136-41.

[13] Campbell, C.F., Chang, A.M., Sease, K.L., et al. (2009). Combining Thrombolysis in Myocardial Infarction risk score and clear-cut alternative diagnosis for chest pain risk stratification. *Am. J. Emerg. Med.*, 27, 37-42.

[14] Cannon, C.P., Weintraub, W.S., Demopoulos, L.A., et al. (2001). TACTICS (Treat Angina with Aggrastat and Determine Cost of Therapy with an Invasive or Conservative Strategy)--Thrombolysis in Myocardial Infarction 18 Investigators. Comparison of early invasive and conservative strategies in patients with unstable coronary syndromes treated with the glycoprotein IIb/IIIa inhibitor tirofiban. *N. Engl. J. Med.*, 344, 1879-87.

[15] Chase, M., Brown, A.M., Robey, J.L., et al. (2007). Application of the TIMI risk score in ED patients with cocaine-associated chest pain. *Am. J. Emerg. Med.*, 25, 1015-8.

[16] Chase, M., Robey, J.L., Zogby, K.E., et al. (2006). Prospective validation of the Thrombolysis in Myocardial Infarction Risk Score in the emergency department chest pain population. *Ann. Emerg. Med.*, 48, 252-9.

[17] Christenson, J., Innes, G., McKnight, G., et al. (2004). Safety and efficiency of emergency department assessment of chest discomfort. *CMAJ*, 170, 1803-7.

[18] Conway Morris, A., Caesar, D., Gray, S., et al. (2006). TIMI risk score accurately risk stratifies patients with undifferentiated chest pain presenting to an emergency department. *Heart,* 92, 1333-4.

[19] Cooney, M.T., Dudina, A.L., Graham, I.M. (2009). Value and limitations of existing scores for the evaluation of cardiovascular risk: A review for clinicians. *J. Am. Coll. Cardiol.*, 54, 1209–27.

[20] Christenson, J., Innes, G., McKnight, D., et al. (2006). A clinical prediction rule for early discharge of patients with chest pain. *Ann Emerg. Med.,* 47, 1-10.

[21] Dagnone, E., Collier, C., Pickett, W., et al. (2000). Chest pain with non-diagnostic electrocardiogram in the emergency department: a randomized controlled trial of two cardiac marker regimens. *CMAJ*, 162, 1561-6.

[22] Dawber, T.R., Meadors, G.F., Moore, F.E. (1950). National Heart Institute, National Institues of Health, Public Health Service, Federal

Security Agensy, Washington, D. C., Epidemiological Approaches to Heart Disease: The Framingham Study. Presented at a Joint Session of the Epidemiology, Health Officers, Medical Care, and Statistics Sections of the American Public Health Association, at the Seventy-eighth Annual Meeting in St. Louis, Mo., November 3, 1950.

[23] de Araujo Goncalves, P., Ferreira, J., Aguiar, C., et al. (2005). TIMI, PURSUIT, and GRACE risk scores: sustained prognostic value and interaction with revascularization in NSTE-ACS. *European Heart Journal*, 26, 865-72.

[24] Diercks, D.B., Hollander, J.E., Sites, F., et al. (2004). Derivation and Validation of a Risk Stratification Model to Identify Coronary Artery Disease in Women Who Present to the Emergency Department with Potential Acute Coronary Syndromes. *Acad. Emerg. Med.,* 11, 630–634.

[25] Douglas, P.S. and Ginsburg, G.S. (1996). The evaluation of chest pain in women. N Engl J Med, 334, 1311–5.

[26] Eagle, K.A., Lim, M.J., Dabbous, O.H., et al. (2004). GRACE Investigators. A validated prediction model for all forms of acute coronary syndrome: estimating the risk of 6-month postdischarge death in an international registry. *JAMA*, 291, 2727-33.

[27] Gale, C.P., Manda, S.O., Weston, C.F., et al. (2009). Evaluation of risk scores for risk stratification of acute coronary syndromes in the Myocardial Infarction National Audit Project (MINAP) database. *Heart*, 95, 221-7.

[28] Garcia-Almagro, F.J., Gimeno, J.R., Villegas, M., et al. (2008). Prognostic value of the Thrombolysis in Myocardial Infarction risk score in a unselected population with chest pain. Construction of a new predictive model. *Am. J. Emerg. Med.,* 26, 439-45.

[29] Geleijnse, M.L., Elhendy, A., Kasprzak, J.D., et al. (2000). Safety and prognostic value of early dobutamine-atropine stress echocardiography in patients with spontaneous chest pain and a non-diagnostic electrocardiogram. *Eur. Heart. J.,* 21, 397– 406.

[30] Goldberg, R.J., O'Donnell, C., Yarzebski, J., et al. (1998). Sex differences in symptom presentation associated with acute myocardial infarction: a population-based perspective. *Am. Heart .J.,* 136, 189–95.

[31] Goldman, L., Cook, E.F., Brand, D.A., et al. (1988). A computer protocol to predict myocardial infarction in emergency department patients with chest pain. *N. Engl. J. Med.,* 318, 797-803.

[32] Goldman, L., Cook, E.F., Johnson, P.A., et al. (1996). Prediction of the need for intensive care in patients who come to the emergency departments with acute chest pain. *N.Engl. J. Med.,* 334, 1498-504.

[33] Goldman, L. and Lee, T.H. (2000). Evaluation of the patient with acute chest pain. *N. Engl. J. Med.*, 342, 1187-1195.

[34] Goldman, L., Weinberg, M., Weisberg, M., et al. (1982). A computer-derived protocol to aid in the diagnosis of emergency room patients with acute chest pain. *N. Engl. J. Med.,* 307, 588-596.

[35] Han, J.H., Lindsell, C.J., Storrow, A.B., et al. (2007). The role of cardiac risk factor burden in diagnosing acute coronary syndromes in the emergency department setting. *Ann. Emerg. Med.,* 49, 145-152.

[36] Henrikson, C.A., Howell, E.E., Bush, D.E., et al. (2003). Chest pain relief by nitroglycerin does not predict active coronary artery disease. *Ann. Intern. Med.,* 139, 979-986.

[37] Hoffmann, U., Nagurney, J.T., Moselewski, F., et al. (2006). Coronary multidetector computed tomography in the assessment of patients with acute chest pain. *Circulation,* 114, 2251-60.

[38] Hollander, J.E., Blomkalns, A.L., Brogan, G.X., et al. (2004). Standardized reporting guidelines for studies evaluating risk stratification of emergency department patients with potential acute coronary syndromes. *Ann. Emerg. Med.,* 44, 589–98.

[39] Hollander, J.E., Chang, A.M., Shofer, F.S., et al. (2009). Coronary computed tomographic angiography for rapid discharge of low-risk patients with potential acute coronary syndromes. *Ann. Emerg. Med.,* 53, 295-304.

[40] Hollander, J.E., Sease, K.L., Sparano, D.M., et al. (2004). Effects of neural network feedback to physicians on admit/discharge decision for emergency department patients with chest pain. *Ann. Emerg. Med.*, 44, 199-205.

[41] Holper, E.M., Antman, E.M., McCabe, C.H., et al. (2001). A simple, readily available method for risk stratification of patients with unstable angina and non-ST elevation myocardial infarction. *Am. J. Cardiol.,* 87, 1008-10.

[42] Jacobs, D.R. Jr., Kroenke, C., Crow, R., et al. (1999). PREDICT: a simple risk score for clinical severity and long-term prognosis after hospitalization for acute myocardial infarction or unstable angina: the Minnesota Heart Survey. *Circulation*, 100, 599–607.

[43] Jaffery, Z., Hudson, M.P., Jacobsen, G., et al. (2007). Modified thrombolysis in myocardial infarction (TIMI) risk score to risk stratify

patients in the emergency department with possible acute coronary syndrome. *J. Thrombosis Thrombolysis*, 24, 137-44.

[44] Jayes, R.L. Jr., Beshansky, J.R., D'Agostino, R.B., et al. (1992). Do patients' coronary risk factor reports predict acute cardiac ischemia in the emergency department? A multicenter study. *J. Clin. Epidemiol.*, 45, 621-6.

[45] Karounos, M., Chang, A.M., Robey, J.L., et al. (2007). TIMI risk score: does it work equally well in both males and females? *Emerg. Med. J.*, 24, 471-474.

[46] Kontos, M.C., Jesse, R.L. (2000). Evaluation of the Emergency Department Chest Pain Patient. *Am. J. Cardiol.*, 85, 32B–39B.

[47] Kushner, F.G., Hand, M., Smith, S.C., et al. (2009). ACC/AHA Guidelines for the Management of Patients With ST-Elevation Myocardial Infarction (Updating the 2004 Guideline and 2007 Focused Update) and ACC/AHA/SCAI Guidelines on Percutaneous Coronary Intervention (Updating the 2005 Guideline and 2007 Focused Update). *Circulation*, 120, 2271-2306.

[48] Lau, J., Ioannidis, J.P., Balk, E.M., et al. (2001). Diagnosing acute cardiac ischemia in the emergency department: a systematic review of the accuracy and clinical effect of current technologies. *Ann. Emerg. Med.*, 37, 453-60.

[49] Lau, J., Ioannidis, J., Balk, E., et al. (2001). Evaluation of Technologies for Identifying Acute Cardiac Ischemia in Emergency Departments. Evidence Report/Technology Assessment Number 26. (Prepared by The New England Medical Center Evidence-based Practice Center under Contract No. 290-97-0019) AHRQ Publication No. 01-E006, Rockville, MD: Agency for Healthcare Research and Quality. May 2001.

[50] Lee, T.H., Rouan, G.W., Weisberg, M.C., et al. (1987). Clinical characteristics and natural history of patients with acute myocardial infarction sent home from the emergency room. *Am. J. Cardiol.*, 60, 219-24.

[51] Limkakeng, A., Gibler, W.B., Pollack, C., et al. (2001). Combination of Goldman Risk and Initial Cardiac Troponin I for Emergency Department Chest Pain Patient Risk Stratification. *Acad. Emerg. Med.*, 8, 696–702.

[52] Lyon, R., Morris, A.C., Caesar, D., et al. (2007). Chest pain presenting to the Emergency Department--to stratify risk with GRACE or TIMI? *Resuscitation*, 74, 90-3.

[53] Manini, A.F., McAfee, A.T., Noble, V.E., Bohan, J.S. (2006). Acute cardiac ischemia time-insensitive predictive instrument predicts exercise

treadmill test outcomes in the chest pain unit. *Am. J. Emerg. Med.,* 24, 375-8.

[54] Manini, A.F., Dannemann, N., Brown, D.F., et al. (2009). Rule-Out Myocardial Infarction using Coronary Artery Tomography (ROMICAT) Study Investigators. Limitations of risk score models in patients with acute chest pain. *Am. J. Emerg. Med.,* 27, 43-8.

[55] Marsan, R.J., Shaver, K.J., Sease, K.L., et al. (2005). Evaluation of a clinical decision rule for young adult patients with chest pain. *Acad. Emerg. Med.,* 12, 26-32.

[56] McCarthy, B.D., Beshansky, J.R., D'Agostino, R.B. et al. (1993). Missed diagnoses of acute myocardial infarction in the emergency department: results from a multicenter study. *Ann. Emerg. Med.,* 22, 579-82.

[57] Miller, C.D., Lindsell, C.J., Khandelwal, S., et al. (2004). Is the Initial Diagnostic Impression of ''Noncardiac Chest Pain'' Adequate to Exclude Cardiac Disease? *Ann. Emerg. Med.,* 44, 565-574.

[58] Morrow, D.A., Antman, E.M., Giugliano, R.P., et al. (2001). A simple risk index for rapid initial triage of patients with ST-elevation myocardial infarction: an InTIME II substudy. *Lancet,* 358, 1571–1575.

[59] Morrow, D.A., Antman, E.M., Snapinn, S.M., et al. (2002). An integrated clinical approach to predicting the benefit of tirofiban in non-ST elevation acute coronary syndromes. Application of the TIMI Risk Score for UA/NSTEMI in PRISM-PLUS. *Eur. Heart J.,* 23, 223-9.

[60] Myocardial Infarction, Task Force for the Redefinition of; Joint ESC/ACCF/AHA/WHF (2007). Universal definition of myocardial infarction. Circulation, 116, 2634-2653.

[61] Panju, A.A., Hemmelgarn, B.R., Guyatt, G.H., et al. (1998). The rational clinical examination. Is this patient having a myocardial infarction? *JAMA,* 280, 1256-63.

[62] Penque, S., Halm, M., Smith, M., et al. (1998). Women and coronary disease: relationship between descriptors of signs and symptoms and diagnostic and treatment course. *Am. J. Crit. Care,* 7, 175–82.

[63] Pollack, C.V., Roe, M.T., Peterson, E.D. (2003). 2002 Update to the ACC/AHA guidelines for the management of patients with unstable angina and non-ST-segment elevation myocardial infarction: implications for emergency department practice. *Ann. Emerg. Med.,* 41, 355-369.

[64] Pollack, C.V. Jr., Sites, F.D., Shofer, F.S., et al. (2006). Application of the TIMI risk score for unstable angina and non-ST elevation acute

coronary syndrome to an unselected emergency department chest pain population. *Acad. Emerg. Med.,* 13, 13-8.

[65] Pope, J.H., Aufderheide, T.P., Ruthazer, R., et al. (2000). Missed diagnoses of acute cardiac ischemia in the emergency department. *N. Engl. J. Med.*, 342, 1163-70.

[66] Pope, J.H., Ruthazer, R., Beshansky, J.R., et al. (1998). Clinical features of emergency department patients presenting with symptoms suggestive of acute cardiac ischemia: a multicenter study. *J. Thromb. Thrombolysis,* 6, 63–74.

[67] Ramsay, G., Podogrodzka, M., McClure, C., et al. (2007). Risk prediction in patients presenting with suspected cardiac pain: the GRACE and TIMI risk scores versus clinical evaluation. *QJM,* 100, 11-8.

[68] Reilly, B.M., Evans, A.T., Schaider, J.J., et al. (2002). Impact of a clinical decision rule on hospital triage of patients with suspected acute cardiac ischemia in the emergency department. *JAMA,* 288, 342-350.

[69] Sabatine, M.S., Antman, E.M., et al. (2003). The thrombolysis in myocardial infarction risk score in unstable angina/non-ST-segment elevation myocardial infarction. *J. Am. Coll. Cardiol.*, 41, 89S-95S.

[70] Sanchis, J., Bodi, V., Nunez, J., et al. (2005). New risk score for patients with acute chest pain, non-ST-segment deviation, and normal troponin concentrations. *J. Am. Col. Cardiol.*, 46, 443-449.

[71] Scirica, B.M., Cannon, C.P., Antman, E.M., et al. (2002). Validation of the thrombolysis in myocardial infarction (TIMI) risk score for unstable angina pectoris and non-ST-elevation myocardial infarction in the TIMI III registry. *Am. J. Cardiol.,* 90, 303-5.

[72] Selker, H.P., Griffith, J.L., D'Agostino, R.B. A tool for judging coronary care unit admission appropriateness, valid for both real-time and retrospective use. A time-insensitive predictive instrument (TIPI) for acute cardiac ischemia: a multicenter study. *Med. Care,* 29, 610-27.

[73] Selker, H.P., Beshansky, J.R., Griffith, J.L., et al. (1998). Use of the Acute Cardiac Ischemia Time-Insensitive Predictive Instrument (ACI-TIPI) To Assist with Triage of Patients with Chest Pain or Other Symptoms Suggestive of Acute Cardiac Ischemia. *Ann. Int. Med.,* 129, 845-855.

[74] Selker, H.P., et al. (1997). An evaluation of technologies for identifying acute cardiac ischemia in the emergency department: a report from a National Heart Attack Alert Program Working Group. *Ann. Emerg. Med.*, 29, 13-87.

[75] Singh, M., Reeder, G.S., Jacobsen, S.J., et al. (2002). Scores for post-myocardial infarction risk stratification in the community. *Circulation,* 106, 2309-14.

[76] Slater, D.K., Hlatky, M.A., Mark, D.B., et al. (1987). Outcome in suspected acute myocardial infarction with normal or minimally abnormal admission electrocardiographic findings. *Am. J. Cardiol.,* 60, 766-70.

[77] Swap, C.J. and Nagurney, J.T. (2005). Value and limitations of chest pain history in the evaluation of patients with suspected acute coronary syndromes. *JAMA,* 294, 2623-9.

[78] Tierney, W.M., Roth, B.J., Psaty, B., et al. (1985). Predictors of myocardial infarction in emergency room patients. *Critical Care Medicine,* 13, 526-31.

[79] Vorlat A., Claeys, M.J., De Raedt, H., et al. (2008). TIMI risk score underestimates prognosis in unstable angina/non-ST segment elevation myocardial infarction. *Acute Cardiac Care,* 10, 26-9.

[80] Walker, N.J., Sites, F.D., Shofer, F.S., et al. (2001). Characteristics and outcomes of young adults who present to the emergency department with chest pain. *Acad. Emerg. Med.,* 8, 703–8.

[81] Weisenthal, B.M., Chang, A.M., Walsh, K.M., et al. (2010). Relation between thrombolysis in myocardial infarction risk score and one-year outcomes for patients presenting at the emergency department with potential acute coronary syndrome. *Am. J. Cardiol.* (ePub available online).

[82] Welch, R.D., Zalenski, R.J., Shamsa, F., et al. (2000). Pretest probability assessment for selective rest sestamibi scans in stable chest pain patients. *Am. J. Emerg. Med.,* 18, 789-792.

[83] Wilson, P.W.F., D'Agostino, R.B., Levy, D., et al. (1998). Prediction of coronary heart disease using risk factor categories. *Circulation,* 97, 1837-1847.

[84] Wood, D., De Backer, G., Faergeman, O., et al., together with members of the Task Force for Prevention of coronary heart disease in clinical practice (1998). Summary of recommendations of the Second Joint Task Force of European and other Societies on Coronary Prevention. *J. Hypertens.,* 16, 1407–1414.

[85] Yan, A.T., Yan, R.T., Jedrzkiewicz, S., et al. (2009). Evaluation of risk scores for risk stratification of acute coronary syndromes. *Heart,* 95, 1019.

[86] Yan, A.T., Yan, R.T., Tan, M., et al. (2007). Risk scores for risk stratification in acute coronary syndromes: useful but simpler is not necessarily better. *Eur. Heart J.*, 28, 1072-8.

In: Chest Pain Causes, Diagnosis and Treatment   ISBN 978-1-61728-112-9
Editor: Sophie M. Weber, pp. 65-95   © 2010 Nova Science Publishers, Inc.

Chapter 3

Body Surface Potential Mapping in the Assessment of Chest Pain

Michael John Daly
Royal Victoria Hospital, Belfast, United Kingdom

Introduction

Body surface potential mapping was first described by Flowers and Horan, as a method to obtain more extensive and precise information than that provided by the standard 12-lead electrocardiogram (ECG) [1]. Although the dipole model for cardiac electrical activity accounts for ~80% of the hearts electrical activity, in reality this electrical field is much more complex and contains multiple areas of positive and negative potential. Thus, body surface mapping allows a more comprehensive representation of cardiac myocyte depolarisation and repolarisation.

Body surface mapping permits correlation of body surface and epimyocardial events: Monro and colleagues successfully demonstrated a correlation between epicardial recordings from temporary pacing wires post-cardiac surgery and surface recordings using a 37-lead ECG [2]. Furthermore, body surface mapping allows detection of events not detectable by the conventional 12-lead ECG. In 1993, Kornreich *et al* compared body surface maps (BSM) in 131 patients with acute myocardial infarction (76 anterior, 32 inferior, 23 posterior) from 159 normal controls using a 120-lead BSM and discriminant function technique (Table 1).

Table 1. BSM variables incorporated into discriminant function analysis achieving sensitivity 96.6% and specificity 100% for the detection of AMI

Variables
ST-T isointegral at 4 electrode points on the lower left anterior chest
ST-T negative area at 2 electrode points on the lower left anterior chest
QRS maximum negative electrode point 11 on the right central chest
Maximum ST-T isointegral over the 64 electrodes
Four quadrants of the ST60ms potential surface
One quadrant of the ST-T negative surface area
Age of the subject

They found that 5/6 (83%) of the leads which optimally classified acute myocardial infarction (AMI) lay beyond the conventional precordial lead-set [3]. In addition, body surface mapping permits both spatial and temporal analysis of the cardiac electrical field, given that each potential recorded at the body surface represents all electrical activity in the thorax at that particular instant [4]. As such, body surface mapping describes the cardiac generator in more complex forms, enabling the development of computational methods and mathematical models to improve our understanding of the relationship between cardiac electrical activity and events recorded at the body surface.

There are many reasons why the 12-lead ECG is suboptimal in the detection of myocardial infarction. Firstly, confounding abnormalities on the 12-lead ECG such as intraventricular conduction disturbances, left ventricular hypertrophy (LVH) and paced rhythms make definitive diagnosis of an acute coronary syndrome (ACS) difficult. Indeed, left bundle branch block (LBBB) and LVH on the initial ECG is associated with much poorer outcomes, probably due to suboptimal risk stratification and delay to treatment [5, 6]. Finally, there are regions of the heart that remain "electrically silent" to the 12-lead ECG due to a lack of leads evaluating these important areas. Currently in its traditional form, the precordial leads (V1 - V6) provide a panoramic view of the electrical activity in the horizontal plane, but are unable to fully assess the anterior wall of the right ventricle or the posterior wall of the left ventricle. Furthermore, the limb leads grouped in the conventional hexaxial system provide a suboptimal view of the cardiac frontal plane, leaving a 60° gap between leads I and II, and a 90° gap between leads III and aVR. This results in under-detection of injury currents originating from the left ventricle's inferior and lateral walls [7].

After decades of focussing urgent treatment on patients with ST elevation, it appears that those with Non-ST elevation myocardial infarction (Non-STEMI) are being mismanaged, despite accounting for an increasing proportion of cardiac admissions. An invasive strategy has been shown to be beneficial for patients with Non-STEMI, especially those with concomitant ST-depression [8]. More rapid detection, triage and treatment are needed for such patients to improve their cardiovascular outcomes. Thus, the European Society of Cardiology published updated guidelines on the acute management Non-STEMI in 2007, highlighting the importance of earlier identification, earlier treatment with anti-platelet, anti-ischaemic and anti-coagulant medications and recommending a more invasive treatment strategy [9]. In terms of earlier identification, primary to the diagnosis of ACS is the initial 12-lead ECG. Following a significant ischaemic event, ECG changes can materialise almost instantaneously, whereas other markers of ischaemia such as cardiac biomarkers can take up to 12 hours to become diagnostic, i.e. troponin T. However, initial decisions regarding prioritisation, i.e. which patient needs further investigation and immediate intervention, can be difficult as ~ 18% of patients with myocardial infarction show no changes on the initial 12-lead ECG [10, 11].

Electrocardiography

In 1856, Kolliker and Müller made the first recording of a cardiac action potential in a frog's heart [12]. However, not until Einthoven's string galvanometer was it possible to adequately summate the electrical output of the human heart [13, 14].

Einthoven's galvanometer consisted of a thin (<3μm) silver-coated quartz filament stretched across a strong magnetic field. When an electric current was passed through the filament, it moved from side-to-side in the magnetic field. Einthoven magnified these small deflections with a projecting microscope, recorded them on a photographic plate moving at a rate of 25mm/s and labelled them *P, Q, R, S* and *T*. This format for recording deflection became the standard and continues to be used to the present day.

The ECG can be recorded using a single electrode connected to an indifferent electrode at zero potential (unipolar) or by using two active electrodes (bipolar). Einthoven used bipolar leads derived from electrodes placed on the left arm (LA), right arm (RA) and left leg (LL) (Figure 1). Through using vector mathematics, he derived the Einthoven triangle – a method of producing three leads (leads I, II and III) on the frontal plane with the heart at its centre. These are the standard limb leads used in electrocardiography. The limb lead voltages (Φ) are obtained as follows:

$$\text{Lead I} = \Phi_{LA} - \Phi_{RA}$$
$$\text{Lead II} = \Phi_{LL} - \Phi_{RA}$$
$$\text{Lead III} = \Phi_{LL} - \Phi_{LA}$$

-   where $I + III = II$

Wilson *et al* were the first to describe a "central terminal" derived from the combination of the three limb leads passed through 5 kOhms of resistance [15]. This provided a zero potential reference point from which a single electrode (V_i) placed on the thorax could be referenced, thus producing a unipolar lead with an absolute value, where:

$$\Phi_W = (\Phi_{LA} + \Phi_{RA} + \Phi_{LL}) / 3$$

A unipolar lead (V_i) can be derived:

$$V_i = \Phi_i - \Phi_W$$

-   where Φ_W = Wilson's Central Terminal

By referencing the potentials of the limb leads from the central terminal, leads VR, VL and VF were produced:

$$VR = \Phi_{RA} - (\Phi_{LA} + \Phi_{LL}) / 2$$
$$VL = \Phi_{LA} - (\Phi_{RA} + \Phi_{LL}) / 2$$
$$VF = \Phi_{LL} - (\Phi_{RA} + \Phi_{LA}) / 2$$

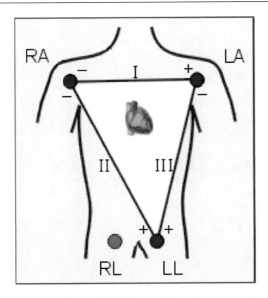

Figure 1. Einthoven Triangle.

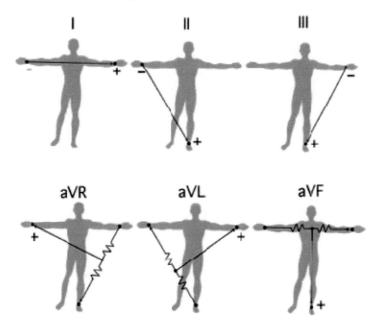

Figure 2. The augmented leads and their associated vectors.

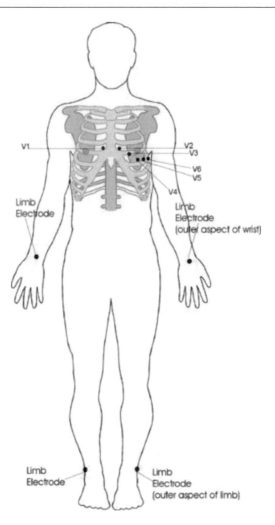

Figure 3. Lead positions of the ECG.

Since the amplitude of these potentials was very small, Goldberger "augmented" these leads by removing the resistance between the extremity and the central terminal [16], thus producing leads aVL, aVR and aVF (Figure 2).

The electrode positions used in the standard 12-lead ECG are shown in Figure 3. They consist of three bipolar leads, located on the right arm, left arm and left leg as described by Einthoven and six unipolar 'precordial' leads $V_1 - V_6$, the position of which is based on the original consensus of the joint committee of the American Heart Association and the Cardiac Society of Great Britain [17].

Lead V_1 is located at the 4th intercostal space at the right margin of the sternum. Lead V_2 at the 4th intercostal space at the left margin of the sternum. Lead V_3 midway between the location of lead V_2 and V_4. Lead V_4 is located at the 5th intercostal space in the mid-clavicular line. Lead V_5 at the 5th intercostal space at the left anterior axillary line. Lead V_6 at the left mid-axillary line at the level of the 5th intercostal space [17]. Although described as the 12-lead ECG, it is clear that this format has only nine actual leads. The discrepancy arises from the fact that the display from this 9-lead configuration produces 12 different outputs: leads I, II, III, avR, avL, avF and $V_1 - V_6$ (as described earlier). This has important implications for future discussion on BSM, and thus from here on any reference to lead numbers (outside that of the standard 12-lead ECG) will correspond to the actual number of electrode leads attached to the thorax.

The Standard 12-Lead ECG in Acute Myocardial Infarction

ST-Elevation Myocardial Infarction

The earliest and most consistent ECG finding with AMI is deviation of the ST-segment [18]. Oppenheimer and Rothschild, as early as 1917 reported on the "electrocardiographic changes associated with myocardial involvement" [19] and in 1920 Pardee reported ST-segment elevation in leads II and III in a patient who had a clinical diagnosis of myocardial infarction [20]. ST elevation myocardial infarction (STEMI) involves total occlusion of a major coronary artery, usually due to acute rupture of a lipid rich, atherosclerotic plaque with subsequent thrombus formation, leading to coronary occlusion, myocardial damage and necrosis. When acute ischaemia is transmural, the overall ST vector is shifted in the direction of the outer epicardial surface. This generally reflects complete occlusion of a major coronary artery, with the leads exhibiting ST-segment elevation reflective of the areas supplied by the occluded artery, e.g. inferior territory ST elevation (leads II, III, aVF) is associated with right coronary artery occlusion, and anteroseptal ST elevation (leads V_1-V_4) corresponding to left anterior descending artery occlusion. Left circumflex territory infarction is less specifically categorised, but lateral ST elevation (leads V_5, V_6, I and aVL) is often associated.

As our understanding of the pathophysiology of endothelial plaque formation and rupture, and thrombus formation has improved so has our ability to treat the condition. Antiplatelet medication such as aspirin [21], clopidogrel [22] and heparin [23] prevent platelet aggregation and adhesion, thus preventing thrombus formation.

It is now well documented that patients suffering STEMI benefit from urgent revascularisation with either thrombolytic agents [24, 27] or primary Percutaneous Coronary Intervention (PCI) and angioplasty [28]. Most European centres use the European Society of Cardiology guidelines (The Minnesota Criteria) of 2 mm ST elevation of the J point in leads $V_1 - V_4$, or 1 mm ST elevation in leads aVL, I, II, aVF, III, V_5 or V_6, as criteria for revascularisation [29]. However, one primary PCI trial used only 1 mm ST elevation in any two adjacent leads as an indication for revascularisation [30] and one trial even used 0.6 mm ST elevation in precordial leads and 0.4 mm in inferior limb leads as an indication for revascularisation [26]. With these improved treatment regimens the mortality for STEMI has fallen from 16% inpatient death in the pre-thrombolysis era, to 4-6% 1-month mortality in the PCI era [25, 26].

Non-ST Elevation Myocardial Infarction

Myocardial infarction without ST elevation on the ECG (Non-STEMI) remains in current focus, as recent data suggests Non-STEMI is increasing in incidence, whereas STEMI appears to be decreasing [31]. ECG changes with Non-STEMI include T-wave inversion, pseudo-normalisation of the T wave and some with no ECG changes at all. However, primary to the diagnosis of Non-STEMI is analysis of the ST segment, namely ST depression. Savonitto et al divided 12,142 patients with ACS in GUSTO IIb into those with T wave inversion (22%), ST elevation (28%), ST depression (35%) and a combination of ST elevation and depression (15%) [32]. Patients with T wave inversion were more likely to have normal coronary arteries (19%), while those with ST depression were more likely to have triple vessel disease (36%). One-month mortality was lowest in those with T wave inversion (1.7%), similar with ST depression or ST elevation (5.1%) and greatest in those with concomitant ST elevation and depression (6.6%). Similar mortality trends were shown at 6-months: 3.4% with T wave inversion, 6.8% with ST elevation, 8.9% with ST depression and 9.1% with ST elevation and depression. This was the first multi-center trial to highlight that patients with ST depression were high-risk and benefited from an earlier invasive strategy with PCI [32].

Furthermore, the degree of ST depression has been shown to confer an increased mortality risk. Kaul *et al*, using information from the PARAGON-A trial on Non-STEMI, showed that 2mm ST depression on admission ECG was associated with a one-year mortality rate of 14.1%, compared with one-year mortality of 6.9% for patients with 1 mm ST depression and 4.4% for those without ST depression [33].

In addition, the GUSTO IV trial (Global Use of Strategies To Open occluded arteries in acute coronary syndrome-IV) showed that patients with ST depression on presentation ECG had an increased probability of death within 30-days, 6-months and one-year when compared to other risk factors for mortality, i.e. troponin T elevation, age, creatinine clearance and blood pressure [34].

Overall, long-term prognosis of Non-STEMI is similar to that of STEMI. In-hospital mortality is higher at 30 days in STEMI patients (7% vs 5%) however, by 6-months mortality rates have almost equalised (13% vs 12%) [32]. Terkelsen *et al* looked at long-term mortality outcomes in ACS patients [35]: one-year mortality in Non-STEMI patients was higher than STEMI patients (31% and 21% respectively). The presence of LBBB on the initial ECG had the worst outcome of all (55% one-year mortality).

Body Surface Potential Mapping

Body Surface Mapping (BSM) is the broad term given to the application of extra electrodes or "non-standard lead sets" over a larger area of the thorax, particularly the high right anterior, posterior and right ventricular territories. The number of electrodes used can range from 15 to 256.

When Waller in the early 19th century described the electrical fields around the heart based on the assumption that the "electromotive force" originated from a dipolar source, the concepts of body surface mapping together with the 12-lead ECG were born [36]. Later, in 1910, Kraus and Nicolai described the spread of cardiac potential on the body surface and asserted that the potentials recorded at the body surface would be similar to those on the surface of the heart beneath (epicardial potentials), nearest to the electrodes [37]. This theory was tested and validated by Barker *et al* when they described the spread of excitation in the ventricles using epicardial electrodes in a patient undergoing a pericardiostomy [38].

The theoretical basis for the 12-lead ECG was on the concept of a single dipole source for all ECG recordings. Were this to be true, then additional leads placed on the thorax would provide little additional information. However, as research into additional lead systems progressed in the early 20th century, it was becoming clear that a single dipolar source for the electrical impulse of the heart was unlikely. This was proposed by Nahum *et al.* who looked at the distribution of the QRS potential at successive instances of time during ventricular excitation and recovery [39]. They noticed that the surface potential field was much more complicated than would be expected from one dipolar source. Subsequently, Nelson presented a study of human thorax potentials recorded from a belt encircling the chest, which recorded multiple ECG recording at the same time [40]. He noticed extremes of potential distribution in differing locations on the chest, which could only be explained if more than one dipole had to be operating at one instant. This was confirmed in further studies, initially on dogs [41] and later healthy humans [42], thus suggesting a more complex electrical model of the heart be adopted. This prompted further investigation into utilising the additional information that the BSM provided over the 12-lead ECG.

In its infancy, body surface mapping was very elaborate and required advances in technology, both instrumentation and computer software, for it to become useful in clinical medicine. Body surface mapping as an entity beyond the 12-lead ECG became more feasible as improved technology allowed researchers to record all relevant surface potentials generated by the cardiac source simultaneously. Initially, the main problem was not with recording the data, but presenting it in a comprehensible fashion. Computer software was primitive and unable to analyse the large quantities of data. Taccardi *et al.* developed a 240-channel instrument with electrodes on the anterior, lateral and posterior chest walls [43]. Each electrode was connected to an amplifier input, which was able to perform analogue to digital conversion with digital tape-recording of the 240 ECGs. Although innovative for the time, it still required 45 minutes for patient preparation and acquisition of signals.

Further instruments were produced all over the world with differing lead numbers and positions. The first commercially available machine was made by Yajima *et al.* in 1983 and was used exclusively in Japan, with similar systems later approved for clinical use in the United States and Europe [44]. Due to research being performed in many centres, there now exist many cardiac mapping systems [45] and a precise mapping technique has not yet been standardised. However, the data analysis and display are quite similar across the board.

Lead Sets

To obtain a truly comprehensive BSM, the number of recording sites needed is much greater than the number of electrodes that can realistically be used [46]. Taccardi's early work used up to 600 electrodes, which is clearly impractical in a clinical setting [42]. Currently, there are a range of BSM recording systems in use, ranging from 15-256 electrodes. The Lux system [47] contains 192 electrodes arranged circumferentially around the torso with the 5th electrode on each strip at the level of V$_2$. There are 16 strips in total, each consisting of 12 electrodes. The Amsterdam, Lux anterior and Lux limited systems are derived from this 192-lead system [45].The Bath system arranges the electrodes equidistantly around the torso. The Helsinki, Brussels and Dalhousie systems are similar, consisting of 120 leads in total with variation in the positioning of the upper anterior and posterior leads. The Montreal system contains 62 electrodes in 10 strips, with 4-7 electrodes on each, while the Japanese system is used predominantly by Japanese research groups. It contains 90 electrodes, each attached separately on the torso surface. Finally, the Parma system consists of 219 electrodes placed in 22 vertical strips, using V$_2$ for attaching electrodes. Interpolation of mapping signals has thus been used in order to obtain a detailed map from a relatively small number of electrodes.

An 80-lead BSM system has been derived based on studies demonstrating the use of interpolation, and also on the premise that the minimum number of electrodes required for the detection of ischaemia is 60 - 120 [46]. Interpolation uses various transformations and prior ECG information to extrapolate data to a larger number of points, thus allowing a reduction in the number of electrodes without any loss of data due to the inherent spatial redundancy of the lead sets. Lux et al developed a 32-lead BSM from his 192-lead BSM system using linear estimation theory interpolation [48] and Barr et al subsequently estimated that 24 optimally placed electrodes were sufficient to produce a BSM of acceptable accuracy [49].

Signal Processing

The recorded electrode signal is initially amplified (using a low frequency filter) and converted from analogue to digital. Recommended sampling rates vary from 0.5-2 kHz, with 1 kHz being adequate for most signals [1]. The digital signal is then filtered to remove baseline wander and mains artefact. Missing data can then be interpolated at this stage and resulting data transferred to a computer for further processing and display.

Data Analysis and Display

Due to the large amount of data recorded from a BSM, summary is essential for interpretation of results. The data can be processed and displayed in scalar waveforms, similar to the current standard 12-lead ECG display format (Figure 4). In this format, one can view each individual electrode as a single beat or as a multitude of beats. This can be useful to examine the posterior regions for Q waves or the right ventricular regions for ST elevation. It also allows the clinician to see QRS morphology and detect conduction delay. The disadvantage with this format, however, is the additional leads presented in this format may add confusion especially to non-cardiology trained physicians. This complexity stems from the requirement to sample multiple ECG channels simultaneously. To overcome this problem, two-dimensional contour maps were developed as a means of simplifying the information into one colour coded output. The commonest types of contour map are isopotential, isointegral and isochrone maps.

Coloured contour maps are described as an area of positive potential (maxima) and an area of negative potential (minima). The maxima are colour coded as red, whereas the minima recorded as blue. A green colour codes for an area of zero potential deflection (isoelectrical). The minimum and maximum refers to the lead with greatest amount of negative or positive deflection respectively. The map is usually displayed as an unwrapped torso surface from the right axilla, with an anterior (or front) section and posterior (back) section [4]. The typical colour contour map is illustrated in Figure 5 with the areas of the flat map which correspond to various territories shown in

Figure 6. A 3-dimensional colour contour display can also be used (Figure 7) that can revolve in multiple planes.

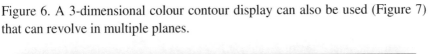

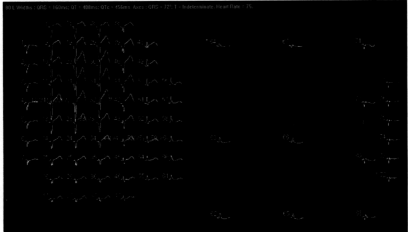

Figure 4. A scalar waveform view of an 80 lead BSM recording of an Acute Anterior ST Elevation Myocardial Infarction. Note the ST segment elevation in the high anterior leads (20, 21, 22, 30, 31, 32), with reciprocal ST depression in the Posterior Leads (62, 65, 68).

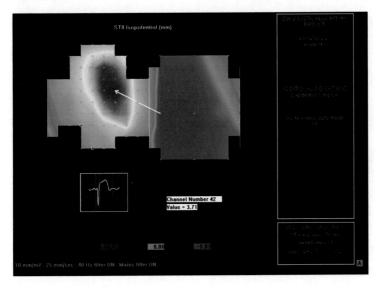

Figure 5. A colour contour mapping display of the same patient in Figure 4. Note the high anterior ST elevation (as highlighted by the red maxima) with posterior ST depression (blue area).

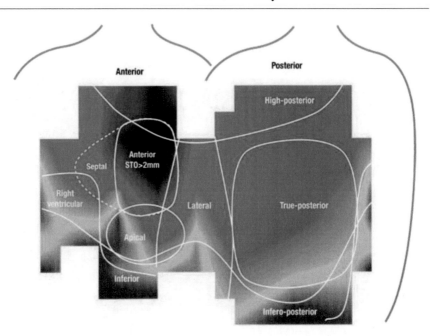

Figure 6. Flat map indicating corresponding areas of myocardium.

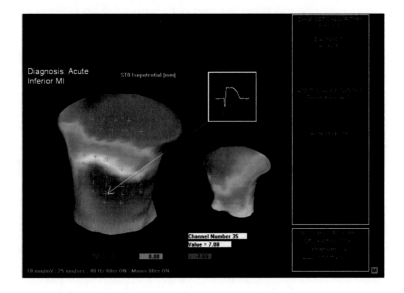

Figure 7. A 3-Dimensional torso representation of an inferior ST elevation MI with ST elevation (red maxima) over the inferior part of the torso.

Isopotential Maps

Colour contour maps can be displayed in a variety of formats. The simplest to appreciate and interpret are isopotential maps, which are the most commonly used in clinical practice These are created by plotting the potentials recorded at each surface electrode for a given time point of the cardiac cycle with contour lines joining points of equal potential. The simplest means of analysis is by direct visual inspection and pattern recognition, similar to that used in 12-lead ECG analysis. The height of the lead potential at the beginning of the ST segment (ST0 or J point) is very important in the diagnosis of myocardial ischaemia. Thus, the ST0 of each lead displayed as a colour contour map can rapidly diagnose infarctions that have evidence of ST elevation and/or depression (Figure 6). Additional Isopotential Maps can be recorded at the ST60 point (60 ms after the J point) or the ST100 (100 ms after the J point) which may be used to confirm repolarisation patterns and look for ST depression.

Isointegral Maps

Another possibility for contour map display is by calculating the summation of potentials for each surface electrode over a particular time period. Integration (area under the curve) over this particular time segment produces an isointegral map (Figure 8), e.g. the QRS isointegral map can be obtained by summation of potentials from each instant from the initial deflection of the QRS to the QRS offset. Similarly the ST-T isointegral map can be determined by the summated area of the ST0 segment to the end of the T wave. The area produced by isointegral maps has the advantage of creating one single map that represents a large period of the cardiac cycle. The QRS isointegral map is used mainly in revealing areas of old MI by showing large negative areas of the QRS (indicating a large Q wave). The ST-T isointegral map can detect subtle changes in the deflections of the T-wave. This can highlight an area which indicates infarction, often revealed as negative T wave deflections. This may be especially important in diagnosing MI in patients where there is no obvious change in the ST segment initially.

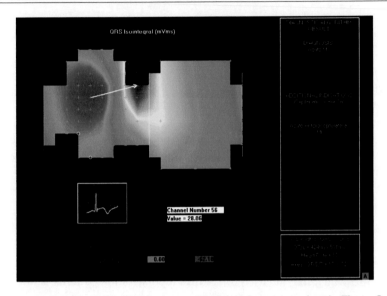

Figure 8. An example of the QRS isointegral BSM of the same patient in Figure 5. Note the differences of the maxima and minima. The colour is produced at the area of the QRS. Positive QRS are red and negative QRS deflections are blue.

For each lead the isointegral value is displayed with contours joining points of the same isointegral value (mVms). One advantage of these maps is that they are averaged over time, thus reducing noise and interference artefact.

Isochronal Maps

An isochrone map displays the spatial variation in a quantity at or in relation to a specific point in time (Isochrone means "same time"; thus isochrone maps indicate events that happen at the same time). The activation time at each lead is defined as either the recorded time of the R wave peak or as the time point at which there is greatest negative rate of change of the QRS voltage (-dP/dt) [1]. This equates to the maximum down slope of the R or S wave. Isochrone maps of depolarisation or repolarisation times are generated using contour plots of the depolarisation or repolarisation time maps. Therefore, in one picture, an isochrone displays the sequence of de-polarisations or repolarisations. The resulting colour contour map highlights the direction of activation wavefronts and may be particularly useful when investigating areas of conduction disturbance.

Clinical Application of the BSM

In the following section, the clinical application of the BSM will be described with particular attention to its use in the assessment of patients presenting with chest pain.

Acute Myocardial Infarction

Kornreich pioneered some of the earliest work on the use of BSM in AMI and its potential application in improving clinical decision making. Using the 120-lead BSM, data from 131 patients with AMI were compared with 159 normal control subjects. The AMI population was stratified according to the location of the ventricular wall motion abnormalities (evidenced by radionuclide imaging) into 76 patients with anterior AMI, 32 patients with inferior AMI and 23 patients with posterior AMI. Using discriminant analysis, the BSM classified 82% of anterior AMI, 93% posterior AMI and 100% inferior AMI. Furthermore, of the 6 leads found to optimally classify AMI, 5 of the 6 lay outside the standard precordial lead positions. Kornreich concluded that "appropriate selection of ECG leads may help remove inconsistencies in current ECG selection criteria and improve comparability of treatment results."[3].

The majority of published work on BSM in AMI has been performed in Belfast, UK. Initial work using the Lux 32-lead BSM system was able to discriminate between AMI and normal controls [50]. McMeechan *et al*, using a 64-lead BSM, compared 194 controls with 101 patients with AMI. They were able to correctly classify 97% of the controls and 74% of the patients with AMI using discriminant function analysis [51]. These findings were confirmed in a subsequent prospective study in a further 48 controls and 59 patients with AMI [52]. In addition, further work was carried out at this centre in 635 patients with ischaemic-type chest pain and 125 normal controls [53]. Of those with chest pain, 325 (51%) had AMI (by WHO criteria); these patients were divided into a training set and a validation set. Multiple logistic regression analysis was performed on the training set to identify the most discriminating variables. These were then incorporated into a model that was tested on the validation set. Using this model, they were able to correctly classify 77% of the controls and 74% of the AMI patients. This was superior to what could be achieved by the 12-lead ECG, as over one-third of patients had a non-diagnostic ECG on presentation.

Right Ventricular and Posterior Myocardial Infarction

Previous studies had demonstrated the importance of right ventricular and posterior leads in the assessment of right ventricular and posterior infarction. In 2000, Menown et al compared the 80-lead BSM with a 16-lead ECG (12-lead ECG with 2 right ventricular leads [V_2R and V_4R] and 2 posterior leads [V_7 and V_9]) to assess whether the improved spatial sampling of the 80-lead BSM could improve detection of right ventricular and posterior infarction in patients with inferior wall AMI [54]. In comparison with prior work, the BSM criteria were based on simple ST elevation criteria using the ST0 isopotential map. Right ventricular involvement was defined as ≥1mm ST elevation in the right ventricular leads of the ECG or BSM. Posterior wall involvement was defined as ≥0.5mm ST elevation on the posterior leads of the ECG or BSM. Infarct size was estimated by serial cardiac enzyme titres. AMI occurred in 173 of 479 patients (36%), with 62 (36%) of those having inferior STEMI. The BSMs in this study were recorded at a median of 1.8hrs post-symptom onset and 8mins after fibrinolytic therapy. Of those with inferior wall AMI, 26 (42%) had right ventricular involvement on the ECG compared with 36 (58%) on the BSM (p = 0.0019). Posterior wall involvement occurred in 6 patients (10%) on the ECG compared with 22 patients (36%) on the BSM (p = 0.00003). Patients with ST elevation on the right ventricular and/or posterior BSMs had a trend towards larger infarct size. Menown et al demonstrated improved classification of patients with inferior wall AMI and right ventricular or posterior wall involvement using the BSM.

Reperfusion of Acute Myocardial Infarction

There have been limited studies comparing the capability of the BSM in assessing reperfusion post-fibrinolytic therapy. Menown et al compared the capability of the 80-lead BSM with the 12-lead ECG at assessing reperfusion in 67 patients treated with fibrinolytic therapy [55]. The patients were divided into a training set and a validation set. The BSM interpretation using discriminant function analysis was compared with ST segment resolution of ≥30% on the 12-lead ECG, with coronary angiography at 90mins post-fibrinolytic therapy the diagnostic gold-standard. Of the 33 patients in the validation set, reperfusion was correctly predicted in 32 (97%) by the BSM, compared with 19 (58%) by the 12-lead ECG.

Acute Coronary Syndrome

Identification and risk stratification of patients with ACS is vital to enable the targeting of those patients who will benefit from further investigations and more aggressive use of pharmacological and interventional strategies. Identification of factors that predict future cardiac events has been carried out in numerous clinical studies and typically includes baseline demographic variables, symptoms, ECG changes and levels of serum cardiac and other biochemical markers [56].

The presentation of AMI appears to be changing. Registry data is highlighting the gradual reduction in STEMI patients presenting to the Emergency Department [57]. Kleiman and White attempted to explain this phenomenon on the grounds of more aggressive aspirin and statin use, and a changing demographic in the patient population (increase age, increased obesity and reduction in smoking) [58]. Non-STEMI now appears to be the mode of presentation to emergency departments and as previously mentioned is associated with increased mortality - those with ST depression on the initial ECG having the worst prognosis [34].

The 12-lead ECG remains the first-line diagnostic investigation in patients with suspected ACS. However, despite significant improvements in other modes of cardiac investigation (Cardiac MRI, CT and Echocardiography), the analysis of the 12-lead ECG still only consists of an assessment of whether the ST segments are elevated or depressed. As mentioned, with BSM there is greater spatial representation of the cardiac electrical field than with the routine 12-lead ECG. This allows for a greater sampling area in terms of detection of electrocardiographic changes not normally perceived by the ECG. This has led to further investigation into improving the detection of AMI through utilising BSM technology. With so many major management decisions based on the 12-lead ECG alone, the question therefore remains: by increasing the number of electrodes would the detection of either ST elevation or depression be increased and thus detection of AMI improved?

The simple addition of V_4R (a right ventricular lead) together with posterior leads V_8 and V_9 (i.e. a 15-lead ECG) has been shown to increase the probability of detecting ST-elevation from 47% to 59% without decrease in specificity [59]. Previous studies have shown the BSM superior in the detection of AMI in the posterior, lateral and inferior regions when compared with the ECG [60, 61]. The main criticism of these early studies was the relatively low numbers of patients and the time delay to procure an adequate BSM recording (ranging from 4 hours - 2 months following presentation), especially when ST changes can resolve following an AMI in a matter of minutes.

The role of BSM has been evaluated in 54 patients presenting with chest pain and ST depression only on their 12-lead ECG [62]. This study compared an optimal BSM model, incorporating multiple isopotential and isointegral variables, with a 12-lead ECG model, incorporating both the number of leads with ST depression and the depth of ST depression. The BSM model improved sensitivity of AMI detection compared with the 12 lead ECG (sensitivity 88% and 38% respectively) whilst maintaining specificity (75%). More recently, comparison of a BSM diagnostic algorithm, developed to aid the physician in BSM interpretation, with a physicians' interpretation of the 12-lead ECG demonstrated that the algorithm improved AMI detection mainly by detecting ST elevation in the posterior and inferior territories [63]. The BSM algorithm detected 10 cases of ST-elevation AMI missed by the physician. Indeed, the 80-lead BSM was superior when compared with the 12-lead ECG to detect AMI in a further study in a pre-hospital setting [64]. For the12-lead ECG, the optimal model included ST elevation, summed ST depression and past history of AMI. BSM criteria for AMI and past history of AMI were included in the optimal model for the BSM. Further research into a novel algorithm using derived epicardial potentials showed even more promising results for the BSM compared with the routine ECG [65].

Chronic Myocardial Infarction

The earlier clinical use of BSM was hampered by the difficulties in applying the electrodes and thus tended to be used in patients recovering from infarction who were therefore more stable. Early work by Flowers [66] in patients with anterior and inferior AMI [67] using departure maps (maps showing differences at an electrode site > 2 standard deviations from the normal population) demonstrated areas of negativity not detected by the 12-lead ECG, i.e. absence of Q waves. This study was performed late in the infarction process, some 13-28 days post index-event.

Vincent et al used 192-lead BSM in 28 patients with previous inferior myocardial infarction and 120 normal controls [68] and also showed Q wave changes not seen on the 12-lead ECG. They concluded that a further 25% of previous myocardial infarctions might not be detected.

Kornreich et al recorded 120-lead BSM from 361 patients (184 normal subjects; 177 patients with myocardial infarction) [69]. Several areas on the

BSM, most of which were located outside the precordial region, contained leads with important discriminant features (mostly ST-T measurements). Using these parameters, they achieved a specificity of 95% and sensitivity of 95% for myocardial infarction detection, compared with a specificity of 95% and a sensitivity of 88% using standard 12-lead ECG parameters.

De Ambroggi *et al* recorded 140-lead isopotential and isointegral maps in 60 patients (30 normal controls, 15 patients with previous inferior myocardial infarction and ECG signs of myocardial necrosis and 15 patients with previous inferior myocardial infarction and no signs of necrosis) [70]. Detection of an abnormal inferior minima in isointegral maps allowed correct classification in 100% of patients with ECG necrosis and 73% of patients without ECG necrosis.

Montague *et al* also performed BSM in patients with Non-STEMI, i.e. non-Q wave myocardial infarction, and detected abnormal Q waves in regions outside the precordial leads of the 12-lead ECG which were associated with significant wall motion abnormalities on ventriculography [71].

Left Bundle Branch Block

Patients with AMI and left bundle branch block (LBBB) have a worse prognosis than those without LBBB and are less likely to receive fibrinolysis, mainly due to difficulties in early diagnosis and uncertainty in distinguishing whether the LBBB is new or longstanding. It is therefore important to optimise the early diagnosis, in order to facilitate prompt treatment. Musso *et al* analysed BSM recorded in patients with LBBB ± AMI and observed lower potential values in patients with LBBB complicated by AMI. Menown *et al* compared QRS and ST-T isointegral maps using an 80-lead BSM system in 22 patients with AMI and LBBB and 19 healthy volunteers with LBBB [53]. In patients with LBBB but no AMI, the loci of the maxima and minima typically reversed positions when comparing the QRS and ST-T isointegral maps, i.e. a vector shift of 180° ± 15°. In contrast, patients with LBBB and AMI showed a reduced vector shift. Subsequently, Maynard *et al* compared validated ECG criteria for LBBB AMI with the BSM in 56 patients with ischaemic-type chest pain and LBBB. Of the 56 patients, 18 had AMI confirmed by cardiac enzyme elevation. Patients with loss of BSM image reversal were significantly more likely to have AMI (odds ratio 4.9, 95% CI: 1.5 − 16.4, p = 0.007). Loss of BSM image reversal was significantly more sensitive (67%) for AMI detection than two previously published 12-lead ECG criteria (17%, 33%) albeit with some loss in specificity (BSM 71%, 12-lead ECG 87%, 97%) [72].

Arrhythmia Diagnosis

BSM has been used in the investigation of various cardiac arrhythmias. Wolf Parkinson White (WPW) syndrome is characterised as attacks of paroxysmal atrial arrhythmia with accelerated atrio-ventricular conduction. In WPW this is due to an additional aberrant connection (bundle of Kent) between the atria and ventricle. Oguri et al. first used BSM to identify the site of an accessory pathway in WPW patients [73]. They were able to divide patients into four distinct groups, indicating the site of the aberrant conduction. This has extremely useful benefits for electrophysiologists planning a procedure such as ablation of the aberrant pathway, in providing information on the location of the accessory pathway.

Cardiac Resynchronisation Therapy

Cardiac resynchronisation therapy (CRT) involves a pacemaker that mechanically resynchronises the contractions of the ventricles by biventricular pacing. Cardiac dyssynchrony is common in heart failure patients, and is normally revealed electrocardiographically as prolonged QRS duration, with LBBB morphology. CRT devices have three leads, one in the atrium, one in the right ventricle, and a final one is inserted through the coronary sinus to pace the left ventricle. CRT devices are shown to reduce mortality and improve quality of life in heart failure patients, however information is lacking as to selecting the optimum patients who will benefit from this device. In a recent study, Shannon et al have shown how BSM criteria could highlight patients who would benefit from CRT, beyond simply looking at QRS duration [74].

Limitations of the BSM

Despite the advantages of the BSM over both the 12-lead and 16-lead ECG, there remains a significant number of AMIs undiagnosed at presentation. Although the BSM permits a better description of the cardiac generator, the potentials measured do not take into account the effects of the thoracic volume conductor. Inverse electrocardiology, i.e. electrocardiographic imaging (ECGI), aims to provide detailed spatial and temporal information on cardiac electrical activity from recorded signals, usually in the form of body surface recordings [75].

Despite the evidence discussed, body surface mapping has largely been used as a research tool and as such, has not gained acceptance into a clinical context. BSM harness application, whilst significantly improved from earlier systems, is occasionally problematic in patients at the extremes of torso size, in particular women with large breasts. In addition, there remains a lack of consensus amongst research groups regarding the optimum number and configuration of electrodes. Lastly, with regard to epicardial potential derivation, it would be ideal to use a tailored thoracic volume conductor model that would take account of the individual patient's body habitus in its use of measured surface potentials and the inverse solution calculation. There is ongoing work in this area.

Conclusion

There is a need for more sensitive and specific screening tests and methods of diagnosing coronary artery disease. BSM may be a feasible and intuitive alternative tool to the 12-lead ECG [76]. The multiple electrodes used sample electrical activity of the cardiac muscle, almost in its entirety. The method of application of the vest requires minimal prerequisite training and is user friendly. Analytic software has been recently tailored to make it more easily accessible to frontline staff. Furthermore, myocardial infarction-ischemia detected by BSM has been shown to consistently correlate with angiographic findings. Work is ongoing in the field of using BSM to detect transient myocardial ischemia, making it more applicable to the legions of patients who present daily to the Emergency Departments and general practitioner (GP) surgeries with chest pain of uncertain aetiology. Preliminary studies have been promising. In their 2007 review of the 12-lead ECG, the American Heart Association Electrocardiography and Arrhythmias Committee, Council on Clinical Cardiology; the American College of Cardiology Foundation; and the Heart Rhythm Society [77] acknowledged the contribution of additional leads in the diagnosis of acute infarction but cited the complexity of BSM as an impediment to replacing the 12-lead ECG. Given the advancement in making the acquisition and analysis of these maps less unwieldy, it might soon be time to re-evaluate the role of BSM in the assessment of the patient with coronary artery disease. The way forward might be best paved with electrodes.

References

[1]   Flowers NC, Horan LG. Body Surface Potential Mapping. In: Zipes DP, Jalife J, editors. Cardiac electrophysiology: From Cell to Bedside. Philadelphia: Saunders, 1995: 1049-67

[2]   Monro DM, Bones PJ, Stanbridge RD et al. Comparison of epicardial and body surface ECG potentials in man. *Cardiovasc Res* 1986;20:201-207

[3]   Kornreich F, Montague TJ, Rautaharju PM. Body surface potential mapping of ST segment changes in acute myocardial infarction. Implications for ECG enrolment criteria for thrombolytic therapy. *Circulation* 1993;87:773-782

[4]   Riddell JW. Determination of myocardial injury by reconstructing epicardial signals from a non-invasive multi-channel electrocardiograph. MD Thesis (2004), Faculty of Medicine, Queen's University Belfast.

[5]   Stenestrand U, Tabrizi F, Lindback J, Englund A, Rosenqvist M, Wallentin L. Comorbidity and myocardial dysfunction are the main explanations for the higher 1-year mortality in acute myocardial infarction with left bundle-branch block. *Circulation* 2004; 110(14):1896-1902.

[6]   Stephenson K, Skali H, McMurray JJ, Velazquez EJ, Aylward PG, Kober L, Van De Werf F, White HD, Pieper KS, Califf RM, Solomon SD, Pfeffer MA. Long-term outcomes of left bundle branch block in high-risk survivors of acute myocardial infarction: the VALIANT experience. *Heart Rhythm* 2007;4(3):308-313.

[7]   Sgarbossa EB, Barold SS, Pinski SL, et al. Twelve-lead electrocardiogram: the advantages of an orderly frontal lead display including lead –aVR. *J Electrocardiol* 2004;37:141-147

[8]   Diderholm E, Andren B, Frostfeldt G, et al. ST depression in ECG at entry indicates severe coronary lesions and large benefits of an early invasive treatment strategy in unstable coronary artery disease; the FRISC II ECG substudy. *Eur Heart J* 2002;23:41-49

[9]   Bassand JP, Hamm CW, Ardissino D, Boersma E, Budaj A, Fernandez-Aviles F, Fox KA, Hasdai D, Ohman EM, Wallentin L, Wijns W.

Guidelines for the diagnosis and treatment of non-ST-segment elevation acute coronary syndromes. *Eur Heart J* 2007;28(13):1598-1660.

[10] Granger CB, Goldberg RJ, Dabbous O, et al. Predictors of hospital mortality in the global registry of acute coronary events. *Arch Intern Med* 2003;163:2345-2353

[11] Hamm C. Acute coronary syndrome: the struggle for the best in risk stratification and therapy. *Eur Heart J* 2002;23:1074-1075

[12] Kolliker A and Muller H. Nachweis der negativen Schwankung des Muskelstromes am naturlich sich contrahiereden Muaskel. *Verhandl d Phys Med Gesellsch* 1856;6:528-533. Cited by Mirvis DM. 1988. *Body Surface Electrocardiographic Mapping*. Kluwer Academic Publishers, chapter History of Electrocadiographic Leads.

[13] Einthoven W. Un nouveau galvanometer. *Arch néerl des Sciences Exact Nat* série 1901;2(6):625-633. Cited by Snellen HA. 1995. *Willem Einthoven: father of electrocardiography*, Kluwer Academic Publishers, Dordrecht.

[14] Einthoven W. *Herinneringsbundel*. Leiden: Eduard Ijdo. 1902 Cited by Snellen HA. 1995. *Willem Einthoven: father of electrocardiography*, Kluwer Academic Publishers, Dordrecht.

[15] Wilson FN, Macleod AG, Barker PS. Potential variations produced by the heart beat at the apices of Einthoven's triangle. *Am Heart J* 1931;7:207-11.

[16] Goldberger E. A simple, indifferent electrocardiographic electrode of zero potential and a technique of obtaining augmented, unipolar extremity leads. *Am Heart J* 1942;23: 483-492.

[17] Barnes AR, Pardee HEB, White PD, Wilson FN, Wolferth CC, and Committee of the American Heart Association for the Standardization of Precordial Leads. Standardization of precordial leads: Supplementary report. *American Heart Journal* 1938;15(2):235-239.

[18] Van De Werf F, Bax J, Betriu A, Blomstrom-Lundqvist C, Crea F, Falk V, Filippatos G, Fox K, Huber K, Kastrati A, Rosengren A, Steg PG, Tubaro M, Verheugt F, Weidinger F, Weis M, Vahanian A, Camm J, De CR, Dean V, Dickstein K, Filippatos G, Funck-Brentano C, Hellemans I, Kristensen SD, McGregor K, Sechtem U, Silber S, Tendera M, Widimsky P, Zamorano JL, Silber S, Aguirre FV, Al-Attar N, Alegria E, Andreotti F, Benzer W, Breithardt O, Danchin N, Di MC, Dudek D, Gulba D, Halvorsen S, Kaufmann P, Kornowski R, Lip GY, Rutten F. Management of acute myocardial infarction in patients presenting with persistent ST-segment elevation: the Task Force on the Management of

ST-Segment Elevation Acute Myocardial Infarction of the European Society of Cardiology. *Eur.Heart J* 2008;29(23): 2909-2945.

[19] Oppenheimer BS, Rothschild MA. Electrocardiographic changes associated with myocardial involvement. *JAMA* 1917;69: 429.

[20] Pardee HEB. An electrocardiographic sign of coronary artery obstruction. *Arch. Int. Med* 1920;26:244-257.

[21] ISIS-2 (Second International Study of Infarct Survival) Collaborative Group 1988. Randomised trial of intravenous streptokinase, oral aspirin, both, or neither among 17,187 cases of suspected acute myocardial infarction: ISIS-2. *Lancet*, 2, (8607) 349-360.

[22] Yusuf S, Zhao F, Mehta SR, Chrolavicius S, Tognoni G, Fox KK. Effects of clopidogrel in addition to aspirin in patients with acute coronary syndromes without ST-segment elevation. *N Eng J Med* 2001;345(7): 494-502.

[23] Gruppo Italiano per lo Studio della Sopravvivenza nell'Infarto Miocardico. GISSI-2: a factorial randomised trial of alteplase versus streptokinase and heparin versus no heparin among 12,490 patients with acute myocardial infarction. *Lancet* 1990;336(8707): 65-71

[24] Silber S, Albertsson P, Aviles FF, Camici PG, Colombo A, Hamm C, Jorgensen E, Marco J, Nordrehaug JE, Ruzyllo W, Urban P, Stone GW, Wijns W. Guidelines for percutaneous coronary interventions. The Task Force for Percutaneous Coronary Interventions of the European Society of Cardiology. *Eur Heart J* 2005;26(8): 804-847.

[25] Armstrong PW, Granger CB, Adams PX, Hamm C, Holmes D, O'Neill WW, Todaro TG, Vahanian A, Van De Werf F. Pexelizumab for acute ST-elevation myocardial infarction in patients undergoing primary percutaneous coronary intervention: a randomized controlled trial. *JAMA* 2007;297(1): 43-51.

[26] Assessment of the Safety and Efficacy of a New Treatment Strategy with Percutaneous Coronary Intervention (ASSENT-4 PCI) investigators. Primary versus tenecteplase-facilitated percutaneous coronary intervention in patients with ST-segment elevation acute myocardial infarction (ASSENT-4 PCI): randomised trial. *Lancet* 2006;367(9510): 569-578.

[27] Fibrinolytic Therapy Trialists' (FTT) Collaborative Group. Indications for fibrinolytic therapy in suspected acute myocardial infarction: collaborative overview of early mortality and major morbidity results from all randomised trials of more than 1000 patients. *Lancet*, 1994;343(8893): 311-322.

[28] Keeley EC, Boura JA, Grines CL. Primary angioplasty versus intravenous thrombolytic therapy for acute myocardial infarction: a quantitative review of 23 randomised trials. *Lancet* 2003;361(9351): 13-20.

[29] Van De Werf F, Ardissino D, Betriu A, Cokkinos DV, Falk E, Fox KA, Julian D, Lengyel M, Neumann FJ, Ruzyllo W, Thygesen C, Underwood SR, Vahanian A, Verheugt FW, Wijns W. Management of acute myocardial infarction in patients presenting with ST-segment elevation. The Task Force on the Management of Acute Myocardial Infarction of the European Society of Cardiology. *Eur Heart J* 2003;24(1): 28-66.

[30] Gyongyosi M, Domanovits H, Benzer W, Haugk M, Heinisch B, Sodeck G, Hodl R, Gaul G, Bonner G, Wojta J, Laggner A, Glogar D, Huber K. Use of abciximab prior to primary angioplasty in STEMI results in early recanalization of the infarct-related artery and improved myocardial tissue reperfusion - results of the Austrian multi-centre randomized ReoPro-BRIDGING Study. *Eur Heart J* 2004;25(23): 2125-2133.

[31] Kleiman NS, White HD. The declining prevalence of ST elevation myocardial infarction in patients presenting with acute coronary syndromes. *Heart* 2005;91(9): 1121-1123.

[32] The Global Use of Strategies to Open Occluded Coronary Arteries (GUSTO) IIb Investigators. A comparison of recombinant hirudin with heparin for the treatment of acute coronary syndromes. *N Engl J Med* 2006;335(11): 775-782.

[33] Kaul P, Fu Y, Chang WC, Harrington RA, Wagner GS, Goodman SG, Granger CB, Moliterno DJ, Van De Werf F, Califf RM, Topol EJ, Armstrong PW. Prognostic value of ST segment depression in acute coronary syndromes: insights from PARAGON-A applied to GUSTO-IIb. PARAGON-A and GUSTO IIb Investigators. PlateletIIb/IIIa Antagonism for the Reduction of Acute Global Organization Network. *J.Am.Coll.Cardiol.*, 2001;38(1): 64-71.

[34] Westerhout CM, Fu Y, Lauer MS, James S, Armstrong PW, Al-Hattab E, Califf RM, Simoons ML, Wallentin L, Boersma E. Short- and long-term risk stratification in acute coronary syndromes: the added value of quantitative ST-segment depression and multiple biomarkers. *J.Am.Coll.Cardiol* 2006;48(5): 939-947.

[35] Terkelsen CJ, Lassen JF, Norgaard BL, Gerdes JC, Jensen T, Gotzsche LB, Nielsen TT, Andersen HR. Mortality rates in patients with ST-elevation vs. non-ST-elevation acute myocardial infarction: observations from an unselected cohort. *Eur.Heart J* 2005;26(1): 18-26.

[36] Waller AD. A demonstration in man of electromotive changes accompanying the heart's beat. *J Physiol (Lond.)* 1887;8:229-34

[37] Sridharan MR, Horan LG. History of body surface electrocardiographic mapping. In: Mirvis DM ed. Body Surface Electrocardiographic Mapping. Kluwer Academic Publishers, 1988.

[38] Barker PS, Macleod AG, Alexander J. The excitatory process observed in the human heart. *Am Heart J* 1930;5:720-744

[39] Nahum LH, Mauro A, Chernoff HM, Sikand RS. Instantaneous equipotential distribution on surface of the human body for various instants in the cardiac cycle. *J Appl.Physiol* 1951;3(8): 454-464.

[40] Nelson CV. Human thorax potentials. *Ann N Y Acad Sci.* 1957;65:1014-1050

[41] Taccardi B. Distribution of Heart Potentials on Dog's Thoracic Surface. *Circ Res* 1962;XI:862-869

[42] Taccardi B. Distribution of heart potentials on the thoracic surface of normal human subjects. *Circ Res* 1963;12:341-352

[43] Taccardi B, De Ambroggi L, Viganotti C. Body-surface mapping of heart potentials. In: The Theoretical Basis of Electrocardiology, edited by Nelson CV, Geselowitz D. Oxford, Clarendon Press 1976 p436-466.

[44] Yajima K, Kinoshita S, Tanaka H, Ihara T, Furukawa T. Body surface potential mapping system equipped with a microprocessor for the dynamic observation of potential patterns. Medical and Biological Engineering and Computing 1983;21: 83-90.

[45] Hoekema R, Uijen GJH, van Oosterom A. On selectring a body surface mapping procedure. *J Electrocardiol* 1999;32:93-101

[46] Maynard S. Use of body surface mapping to aid the diagnosis of myocardial infarction and ischaemia. 2001 MD Thesis, Faculty of Medicine, Queen's University of Belfast.

[47] Lux RE, Smith R, Abildskov J. Limited lead selection for estimating body surface potentials in electrocardiography. IEEE BME 1978;25:270

[48] Lux RL, Burgess MJ, Wyatt RF, et al. Clinically practical lead systems for improved electrocardiography: comparison with precordial grids and conventional lead systems. *Circulation* 1979;59:356-363

[49] Barr RC, Spach MS, Herman-Giddens GS. Selection of the number and positions of measuring locations for electrocardiography. *IEEE Trans.Biomed.Eng* 1971;18(2): 125-138.

[50] Cullen CM. Body Surface Mapping in the Diagnosis of Acute Myocardial Infarction. 1995 MD Thesis, Faculty of Medicine, Queen's University Belfast.

[51] McMeechan SR, Cullen CM, MacKenzie G, et al. Discriminant function analysis of body surface potential maps in acute myocardial infarction. *J Electrocardiol* 1994;24(Suppl):117-120

[52] McMeechan SR, MacKenzie G, Allen J, et al. Body surface ECG potential maps in acute myocardial infarction. *J Electrocardiol* 1995;28(Suppl):184-90

[53] Menown IBA, Allen J, Anderson JM, et al. Body surface mapping for early diagnosis of acute myocardial infarction with left bundle branch block. *J Am Coll Cardiol* 1998;31(Suppl):229A

[54] Menown IB, Allen J, Anderson JM, et al. Early diagnosis of right ventricular or posterior infarction associated with inferior wall left ventricular acute myocardial infarction. *Am J Cardiol* 2000;85:934-938

[55] Menown IB, Allen J, Anderson JM, et al. Noninvasive assessment of reperfusion after fibrinolytic therapy for acute myocardial infarction. *Am J Cardiol* 2000;86:736-41

[56] Granger CB, Goldberg RJ, Dabbous O, Pieper KS, Eagle KA, Cannon CP, Van De Werf F, Avezum A, Goodman SG, Flather MD, Fox KA. Predictors of hospital mortality in the global registry of acute coronary events. *Arch.Intern.Med.* 2003;163(19): 2345-2353.

[57] Dauerman HL, Lessard D, Yarzebski J, Furman MI, Gore JM, Goldberg RJ. Ten-year trends in the incidence, treatment, and outcome of Q-wave myocardial infarction. *Am.J Cardiol.*, 2000;86(7): 730-735.

[58] Kleiman NS, White HD. The declining prevalence of ST elevation myocardial infarction in patients presenting with acute coronary syndromes. *Heart* 2005;91(9): 1121-1123.

[59] Sgarbossa EB, Birnbaum Y, Parillo JE, et al. Electrocardiographic diagnosis of acute myocardial infarction: Current concepts for the clinician. *Am Heart J* 2001;141:507-517

[60] Sugiyama S, Wada M, Sugenoya JI, Toyoshima H, Toyama J, Yamada K. Diagnosis of right ventricular infarction: experimental study through the use of body surface isopotential maps. *Am.Heart J* 1977;94(4): 445-453.

[61] Yamada K, Toyama J, Sugenoya J, Wada M, Sugiyama S. Body surface isopotential maps. Clinical application to the diagnosis of myocardial infarction. *Jpn.Heart J* 1978;19(1): 28-45.

[62] Menown IB, Allen J, Anderson JM, Adgey AA. ST depression only on the initial 12-lead ECG: early diagnosis of acute myocardial infarction. *Eur.Heart J* 2001;22(3): 218-227.

[63] McClelland AJ, Owens CG, Menown IB, Lown M, Adgey AA. Comparison of the 80-lead body surface map to physician and to 12-lead electrocardiogram in detection of acute myocardial infarction. *Am.J.Cardiol* 2003;92(3): 252-257.

[64] Owens CG, McClelland AJ, Walsh SJ, Smith BA, Tomlin A, Riddell JW, Stevenson M, Adgey AA. Prehospital 80-Lead mapping: does it add significantly to the diagnosis of acute coronary syndromes? *J.Electrocardiol* 2004;37 (Suppl): 223-232.

[65] Owens C, McClelland A, Walsh S, Smith B, Adgey J. Comparison of value of leads from body surface maps to 12-lead electrocardiogram for diagnosis of acute myocardial infarction. *Am.J Cardiol* 2008;102(3): 257-265.

[66] Flowers NC, Horan LG, Johnson JC. Anterior infarctional changes occurring during mid and late ventricular activation detectable by surface mapping techniques. *Circulation* 1976;54:906-913

[67] Flowers NC, Horan LG, Sohi GS, et al. New evidence for inferoposterior myocardial infarction on surface potential maps. *Am J Cardiol* 1976;38:576-581

[68] Vincent GM, Abildskov JA, Burgess MJ, et al. Diagnosis of old inferior myocardial infarction by body surface isopotential mapping. *Am J Cardiol* 1977;39:510-515

[69] Kornreich F, Rautaharju PM, Warren J, et al. Identification of best electrocardiographic leads for diagnosing myocardial infarction by statistical analysis of body surface potential maps. *Am J Cardiol* 1985;56:852-856

[70] de Ambroggi L, Bertoni T, Rabbia C, et al. Body surface potential maps in old inferior myocardial infarction. Assessment of diagnostic criteria. *J Electrocardiol* 1986;19:225-234

[71] Montague TJ, Johnstone DE, Spencer CA, et al. Non-Q wave acute myocardial infarction: body surface potential map and ventriculographic patterns. *Am J Cardiol* 1986;58:1173-1180

[72] Maynard SJ, Menown IB, Manoharan G, et al. Body surface mapping improves early diagnosis of acute myocardial infarction in patients with chest pain and left bundle branch block. *Heart* 2003;89:998-1002

[73] Oguri, H, Wada M, Niimi N, Toyama J, Yamada K. An experimental study of the WPW syndrome-relationship between body surface maps and the preexcitation area of the epicardium. *Adv.Cardiol.*, 1978;21: 31-35.

[74] Shannon J, Navarro CO, McEntee T, Riddell G, Adgey JA, Lau EW. An early phase of slow myocardial activation may be necessary in order to benefit from cardiac resynchronization therapy. *J Electrocardiol* 2008;41(6): 531-535.

[75] Oster HS, Taccardi B, Lux RL, et al. Noninvasive electrocardiographic imaging: reconstruction of epicardial potentials, electrograms, and isochrones and localization of single and multiple electrocardiac events. *Circulation* 1997;96:1012-24

[76] Robinson MR, Curzen N. Electrocardiographic Body Surface Mapping: Potential Tool for the Detection of Transient Ischaemia in the 21st Century? *Ann Noninvasive Electrocardiol* 2009;14(2):201-210

[77] Kligfield P, Gettes LS, Bailey JJ, et al. Recommendations for the standardization and interpretation of the electrocardiogram: Part I: The electrocardiogram and its technology a scientific statement from the American Heart Association Electrocardiography and Arrhythmias Committee, Council on Clinical Cardiology; the American College of Cardiology Foundation; and the Heart Rhythm Society endorsed by the International Society for Computerized Electrocardiology. *J Am Coll Cardiol* 2007;49:1109–1127.

In: Chest Pain Causes, Diagnosis and Treatment   ISBN 978-1-61728-112-9
Editor: Sophie M. Weber, pp. 97-118   © 2010 Nova Science Publishers, Inc.

Chapter 4

The Diagnostic Approach to the Cardiac Patient with Chest Pain

Zehra Jaffery and Arthur G. Grant
Department of Cardiology,
Ochsner Medical Institution, New Orleans, LA, USA

"It is the province of knowledge to speak and it is the privilege of wisdom to listen"- *Oliver Wendel Holmes*

Chest pain has a wide differential diagnosis. It is well recognized as a common presentation of acute coronary ischemia. Despite availability of multiple diagnostic modalities for evaluation of chest pain, the rate of missed myocardial infarction ranges from 2%-10% [1, 2] A patient with known coronary atherosclerotic disease remains at high risk for recurrent coronary events. Nonetheless, similar to any other patient presenting with chest pain, a systematic diagnostic approach is needed. Listening to the patient's description of symptoms is important.

The earliest description of effort angina by William Heberden over 200 years ago still holds true [3]. He described it as *"a disorder of the breast marked with strong and peculiar symptoms. The seat of it, and sense of strangling, and anxiety with which it is attended, may make it not improperly called angina pectoris. Those who are afflicted with it are seized while they are walking and more particularly when they walk soon after eating with painful and most disagreeable sensations in the breast which seems as if it would take their life away if it were to increase or continue. The moment they stand still all this uneasiness vanishes".*

Introduction

Annually 5.8 million emergency department visits occur for the evaluation of chest pain [4]. Among patients evaluated in the emergency department for chest pain, 17%-34% have known coronary artery disease (CAD)[1, 4-6]. Among patients hospitalized for evaluation of chest pain, 49% have a history of known CAD [7]. Among patients undergoing percutaneous coronary interventions (PCI), 6.7% are readmitted within 30 days with chest pain [8]. In patients undergoing coronary arterial bypass surgery, 30% reported frequent episodes of chest pain 2 years post bypass [9]. Current statistics show that an estimated 16, 800, 000 American adults have coronary artery disease [10]. Therefore, chest pain in a patient with known CAD is a commonly encountered clinical scenario.

Patients with a history of myocardial infarction (MI) are a high risk group with approximately one in three presenting with a recurrent MI within 5 years [8, 10]. Owing to the high-risk nature of this patient population, acute coronary syndrome (ACS) is foremost on the differential (Table 1). This chapter discusses the diagnostic approach for three potentially catastrophic diagnoses of chest pain in a patient with CAD.

For any patient presenting with chest pain, the time that should be spent in eliciting a history and examining the patient should be directly proportionate to the clinical condition of the patient. For example, in a clinically unstable patient, therapeutic measures will need to be started even before a thorough history and physical examination has been completed. Physical examination should commence with assessment of vital signs. If the patient becomes hemodynamically unstable during the course of the examination, attention should be turned to resuscitative measures. Prior to ordering diagnostic tests, inherent limitations, benefit and risks should be assessed.

Table 1. Chest pain: Differential diagnosis

Chest pain
Acute coronary syndrome
Pericarditis
Aortic dissection
Hypertrophic cardiomyopathy
Mitral valve proplase
Acute pulmonary embolism
Pulmonary arterial hypertension
Gastroesophageal reflux
Nutcracker esophagus
Costochondritis
Osteoarthritis of the spine
Psychogenic
Peptic ulcer
Acute Pancreatitis
Acute cholecystitis

Acute Coronary Syndrome: History and Physical Examination

Formal investigations have demonstrated that descriptors of chest pain predict ACS weakly or not at all [11, 12]. Variability in history taking leads to poor inter-observer reliability [13.] Despite these limitations, chest pain described as pressure, similar to that of prior MI, accompanied by nausea, vomiting, or diaphoresis or one that radiates to one or both shoulders or arms and increases with exertion has a higher probability of being coronary ischemia [14]. Chest pain that lasts only seconds is rarely indicative of ischemic chest pain, although this has not been demonstrated in studies [15]. The association between coronary ischemia and relief of chest pain with nitroglycerin is unreliable as this can also happen with esophageal causes of chest pain [16, 17].

There is no sign on physical examination that establishes a diagnosis of ACS. In the stable patient, evaluation of vital signs (for example rate and form of an arterial pulse) will provide important information that aids diagnosis and decision making as shown in Table 2. Jugular venous distension in a patient with history suggestive of an ACS may suggest a right ventricular infarct.

Table 2. Chest pain: Value of an arterial pulse

Features of arterial pulse	Significance
Pulses Bisferiens	Hypertrophic cardiomyopathy Aortic stenosis with aortic regurgitation
Pulsus parvus et tardus	Severe aortic stenosis with angina
Collapsing pulse	Severe aortic regurgitation Anemia precipitating angina
Absent left upper extremity pulse	Poor graft flow in left internal mammary artery in a patient with history of coronary bypass
Diminished pulses in lower extremity	Consider upper limb vascular access for angiography

In hemodynamically unstable patients, new onset systolic murmurs in a patient with a recent MI suggest papillary muscle rupture leading to mitral regurgitation or septal wall perforation resulting in a ventricular septal defect.

When it is clear after history and physical examination that the most likely etiology of chest pain in the given patient is coronary ischemia, attention should be directed towards assessing the underlying etiology for coronary ischemia. The most common etiology is rupture of an unstable plaque which can present as an acute MI with complete occlusion (ST segment elevation myocardial infarction) or incomplete occlusion of the underlying coronary artery (Non-ST segment elevation myocardial infarction or unstable angina). Sudden worsening of ischemic symptoms in a cardiac patient with previously controlled angina and known coronary anatomy should prompt work-up of etiologies for worsening symptoms in addition to investigations to assess plaque rupture. Worsening anginal symptoms occur either due to decreased in coronary blood supply, increased demand or both. With a history of PCI or coronary bypass, in-stent restenosis and closure of bypass grafts can lead to recurrent angina.

A detailed medication history should be obtained. For example, intake of over the counter antacids affects absorption of anti-anginal medications and may worsen angina. Factors such as anemia, hyperthyroidism, worsening valvular disease, difficult to control hypertension, new onset arrhythmias and sepsis should be identified.

Acute Coronary Syndrome: Laboratory and other Investigations

In every patient presenting with ongoing chest pain an electrocardiogram (EKG) should be performed immediately. Certain EKG features such as ≥ 1 mm ST segment elevation in 2 contiguous leads, new left bundle branch block suggests an occluded coronary artery. However, it must be remembered that ST segment elevation on an EKG has a wide range of differential diagnosis (Table 3). On the other hand, 50% of patients with ongoing coronary ischemia may not have significant ischemic ST segment changes on an EKG. Always, the current EKG should be compared to previous available tracing. An EKG is of value even in the absence of ongoing symptoms, as signs of recent MI such as new Q waves can be identified. Patients with known CAD and depressed left ventricular function may have implanted intracardiac defibrillators or pacemakers. In an underlying ventricular-paced rhythm, interpreting ischemic ST segment changes reliably is not possible. Underlying coronary ischemia may present as recurrent defibrillator discharges for ventricular tachycardia.

Baseline comprehensive labwork is of value as anemia, electrolyte, endocrine, hepatic and renal abnormalities can be detected. In patients with ACS this affects decision making.

Cardiac troponin (cTnI or cTnT) has emerged as the preferred diagnostic marker for diagnosis of MI [18]. The risk of missing a MI when using a single cTn test upon arrival at the hospital emergency department is 10-15% [19]. American and European guidelines recommend repeat tests for cTn elevation up to 12 hours after the onset of symptoms [18]. Myocardial damage results in elevation of cTn within 6-10 hours after symptom onset and cTn values return to normal in 10-14 days. Other biomarkers, such as creatinine kinase MB (CKMB) fraction and serum myoglobin have different pharmacokinetic profiles (Figure 1). Serum myoglobin is the first biomarker to rise after myocardial damage (within 30-60 min). However, its diagnostic utility is limited owing to low specificity and false positive values seen with rhabdomyolysis, alcohol intake and skeletal muscle trauma [20]. CKMB is also less specific than cTn for diagnosis of myocardial damage. This biomarker rises within 6-8 hours of symptom onset and returns to normal in 12-24 hours [21]. Thus CKMB was traditionally used to diagnose recurrent MI in a patient with recent ACS.

Table 3. Differential Diagnosis of ST-Segment elevation

Description	Associated features	Diagnosis
≥ 1 mm convex upwards ST segment elevation at J point in 2 contiguous leads ≥ 2 mm elevation in V1-V3	ST segment depression in opposite leads	ST segment elevation myocardial infarction
Diffuse concave ST segment elevation	PR depression	Pericarditis
1 mm convex upwards ST segment elevation in 2 contiguous leads	Similar to previous tracing	Ventricular aneurysm
≥ 1 mm concave ST segment elevation	Unchanged from previous tracing	Early repolarization
≥ 1 mm ST segment elevation	Features of left ventricular hypertrophy	Apical hypertrophic cardiomyopathy Left ventricular hypertrophy

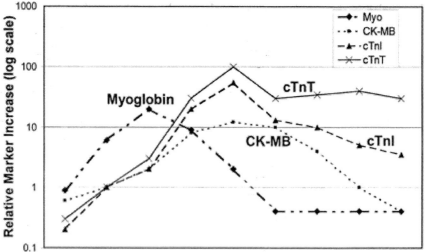

With permission, from Christenson RH, Azzazy HME. Biomarkers of necrosis: past, present and future. In Morrow DA, ed. Cardiovascular Biomarkers: Pathophysiology and Clinical Management. New York: Humana Press, 2006.

Figure 1. Temporal release of myoglobin, CK-MB, cTnI and cTnT.

However, recent guidelines state that recurrent infarction can also be diagnosed by cTn, provided there is a > 20% increase in the value of the second cTn sample [18].

Elevations of cardiac biomarkers reflect myocardial damage but do not suggest mechanism. Elevated cTn is seen with myocardial damage due to ruptured plaque as well as supply demand mismatch seen in anemia, sepsis, hypertensive crisis, decompensated heart failure, acute pulmonary embolism and acute myocarditis [18, 22]. Therefore, biomarker elevation needs to be interpreted within the clinical context and should be remembered as being one of the tools for assessment and management of patients with chest pain.

In addition to myocardial ischemia, ACS is also associated with inflammatory changes and a pro-thrombotic milieu. A number of biomarkers such as C - reactive protein, interleukin-6, brain natriuretic peptide, heart fatty acid-binding protein, glycogen phosphorylase, matrix metalloproteinase-9, myeloperoxidase, CD 40 ligand have been studied for early detection of ACS. Some studies have suggested prognostic value of a multi-marker strategy in patients with chest pain [23-25]. No consensus has yet emerged regarding clinical utility of novel biomarker combinations in patients presenting with chest pain.

When history, physical examination and basic laboratory investigations do not establish or rule out ACS, stress testing has a diagnostic role. It should be performed when the patient is symptom free and an evolving MI has been ruled out [26]. The type of test ordered depends on an individual patient's profile. Exercise EKG is preferred whenever feasible as it also provides an estimation of the patient's functional capacity. If the EKG has baseline ST-T segment changes or is otherwise uninterpretable, then an echocardiogram to visualize wall motion changes with peak stress or nuclear imaging scan to visualize perfusion deficits with stress is recommended. In patients unable to exercise, pharmacological agents such as adenosine, regadenosine or dobutamine can be used as stressors. Nuclear imaging stress test is preferred to stress echocardiogram in those with underlying LBBB, paced rhythm and multiple wall motion abnormalities at rest. Emerging newer modalities of stress testing are cardiac magnetic resonance and positron emission tomography [27, 28]. Data available so far do not suggest an advantage for these modalities, when compared to commonly available modalities of stress testing [29].

The information obtained from the stress test is only as good as the technician performing it and the physician who interprets it. In a patient with known coronary atherosclerosis and atypical chest pain, a stress test assesses the amount of coronary ischemia. The underlying assumption is that, in a patient with chest pain, coronary ischemia is likely responsible for the presenting symptom when a significant amount of coronary ischemia is detected by a stress test. In cardiac patients with angina, stress testing also serves to assess ischemic burden. Adjustment of medications will often suffice for a small area of reversible ischemia while coronary angiography with revascularization is recommended for large areas of reversible ischemia.

Pericarditis

Approximately 5% of patients who present to the emergency department with chest pain are diagnosed with pericarditis [30]. Similar to a non-cardiac patient, pericarditis in the cardiac patient can be caused by trauma to the chest, infection, metabolic imbalance, connective tissues diseases, radiation therapy, malignancy or drugs.

Certain forms of pericarditis are seen only in a cardiac patient. Regional post -infarct pericarditis remains a relatively unknown and under diagnosed condition. Oliva and Mayo first described regional pericarditis 17 years ago [31]. Subsequent case series demonstrate the frequency to vary widely, ranging from 7% to 41%. Incidence is directly related to the time between the onset of symptoms and reperfusion [32, 33]. It is seen in patients 2-4 days post infarct and is associated with transmural MI, anterior wall involvement, left ventricular dysfunction, 3-vessel coronary artery disease and diabetes mellitus [34, 35].

Post cardiac injury syndrome (PCIS) is an inflammatory pericardial and pleural process that occurs 1-4 weeks after cardiac injury but without overt chamber perforation [36]. PCIS was first described in the 1950s in patients undergoing mitral commissurotomy and other cardiac surgeries [37]. PCIS includes two distinct entities, the postmyocardial infarction syndrome (Dressler's syndrome) which occurs after myocardial infarction and the postcardiotomy syndrome which occurs after cardiac surgery or trauma [38]. PCIS has also been seen after intravascular procedures including transvenous pacemaker insertion, AV node ablation and percutaneous coronary intervention. It has been reported in 1.2% to 4.9% of cases after pacemaker insertion and has been described to occur between 1 to 56 days post procedure [39, 40].

Cardiac perforation can present as pericarditis with associated pericardial effusion [41]. This is a life-threatening complication of an invasive cardiac procedure such as percutaneous coronary intervention, electrophysiological ablation etc. It is generally identified during the procedure itself but delayed presentation of cases has been reported. It occurs during the same time frame as PCIS. Clinical presentation is similar to PCIS. A fall in hemoglobin favors the diagnosis of cardiac perforation [36, 42].

Pericarditis: History and Physical Examination

The chest pain of acute pericarditis is retrosternal in location, sudden in onset, and pleuritic in nature. It is often worse with inspiration and when the patient is supine and improves when he or she sits up and leans forward. It often radiates to one or both shoulders [43]. If pericarditis is suspected from the presenting complaint, further questions should be directed to identify the underlying etiology.

Physical examination in cases of suspected pericarditis is directed to verify the diagnosis and identify complications. A careful blood pressure reading should be obtained to look for the presence of pulsus paradoxus (a decrease in systolic arterial pressure of more than 10mm with inspiration) which suggest associated pericardial effusion with a tamponade physiology. The presence of this physical sign increases the likelihood of tamponade physiology (likelihood ratio, 3.3; 95% CI, 1.8-6.3) and absence of this physical sign lowers the likelihood (likelihood ratio, 0.03; 95% CI, 0.01-0.24) [44]. Patients with tamponade are often tachycardic, have elevated jugular venous pressure, muffled heart sounds and may be in cardiogenic shock at presentation. Early detection of tamponade physiology represents a window of opportunity as a lethal outcome in these patients can be avoided by urgent pericardiocentesis.

During auscultation, in patients with suspected pericarditis, one should look for a pericardial friction rub. This is a high-pitched scratchy sound best heard at the left sternal border at end expiration with the patient leaning forward. It can be heard in 85% of patients with pericarditis, at some point during the course of their disease [45]. It has 3 components which correspond to atrial systole, ventricular systole and rapid ventricular filling during ventricular diastole. When a pericardial rub is present, 3 components are discernable in half of the patients, 2 components in a third and 1 component in the remainder [46]. Unlike a pleural rub, this remains audible even when respirations are held [43, 46].

Pericarditis: Investigations

The 12 lead EKG in acute pericarditis classically shows wide spread upward concave ST segment elevation with PR segment depression. The abnormalities evolve through four phases: diffuse ST segment elevation and PR segment depression (stage I); normalization of the ST and PR segments (stage II); widespread T wave inversions (stage III); and normalization of the T waves (stage IV) [47]. While there are no EKG characteristics to diagnose regional pericarditis, two atypical T wave patterns of evolution have been described with a sensitivity and specificity of 77% and 100% respectively [31, 48]. In contrast to MI, which presents with tall peaked T waves that invert within 48 hours and remain inverted for days or weeks post MI regional pericarditis has persistently positive T waves 48 hours after symptom onset and premature gradual reversal of inverted T waves to persistently upright T waves [31, 48].

Transthoracic echocardiography helps in identifying the presence of a pericardial effusion. However, the presence of a pericardial effusion cannot be use as the sole diagnostic criteria for post-infarct pericarditis [49, 50]. Pericardial effusions are common in patients after an MI. They are seen in patients with congestive heart failure when hydrostatic pressure is increased and hemodynamics are impaired and also when there is increased production of interstitial fluid, obstruction of lymphatic drainage or an increase in capillary permeability as in acute pericarditis [51]. If a large to moderate pericardial effusion is seen, evaluation for the presence or absence of tamponade physiology is necessary. Criteria that suggest cardiac tamponade by echocardiography are right ventricular diastolic collapse, right atrial systolic collapse, increase in transmitral inflow E wave velocity more than 25% on inspiration and/or increase in tricuspid inflow E wave velocity greater than 40% on inspiration and inferior vena cava dilatation without collapse on inspiration [52, 53]. If significant mitral flow velocity respiratory flow variation is present without echocardiographic criteria for moderate or a large pericardial effusion, it is appropriate to perform transesophageal echo-cardiography to rule out a loculated effusion causing cardiac tamponade in the appropriate clinical scenario [54].

Other laboratory investigations commonly ordered are tailored to the clinical scenario. A chest radiograph can identify mediastinal pathology. A basic metabolic panel rules out uremia as a cause. Serum C-reactive protein, erythrocyte sedimentation rate, autoimmune profile and microbiological investigations are other commonly ordered tests. The clinical profile of the presenting patient should guide the number and type of investigations ordered.

Acute Aortic Dissection:

Chest pain can be the presenting symptom of acute thoracic aortic dissection (AAD), which is one of the most common and serious diseases of the aorta, and carries a high morbidity and mortality rate when it is not recognized and treated promptly. If left untreated, mortality from AAD rises by 1% to 1.4% per hour, leading to a 68% mortality rate within 48 hours [55], [56]. The aortic wall has 3 layers from inside out: intima, media and adventitia. In AAD a tear in the intima leads to passage of blood into the space between the intima and adventitia with creation of a false lumen. If a patient with aortic dissection presents less than 2 weeks from symptom onset, it is defined as an acute dissection. Predisposing factors for acute aortic dissection (AAD) include hypertension, bicuspid aortic valve, coarctation of the aorta, Marfan syndrome, Ehlers-Danlos syndrome, Turner syndrome, giant cell arterits, pregnancy, cocaine use and trauma. In the patient with known coronary atherosclerosis, recent intra aortic catheterization and cardiac surgery (particularly aortic valve or aortic root replacement) increases the risk for AAD.

There are two similar clinical entities worth mentioning: intramural hematoma (IMH) and penetrating aortic ulcer (PAU). In patients suspected of AAD, the prevalence of IMH ranges between 4% to 28% [57]. IMH has been considered a variant or precursor of aortic dissection with no entry tear or false lumen flow. A hematoma forms within the aortic wall as a result of hemorrhage of the vasa vasorum (blood vessels supplying the aortic wall) or, less commonly, an intimal fracture of an atherosclerotic plaque. The clinical presentation is similar to that of AAD, with a conversion rate of 30% to 40% into a typical dissection [58, 59]. When compared to patients with AAD, these patients are older and have a higher prevalence of female sex and hypertension [60].

PAU refers to a condition where there is an ulceration of atherosclerotic aortic plaques, usually in the descending thoracic or abdominal aorta. These lesions can lead to penetration into the intimal borders and into the media, resulting in an IMH or can dissect along the extent of the aorta, resulting in classic AAD.

Traditionally, clinical diagnosis of AAD has been inaccurate. Only 0.003% of patients presenting to an emergency department with acute back, chest or abdominal pain are eventually diagnosed with AAD [61]. In patients presenting with dissection, physicians correctly suspected the diagnosis in as few as 15% to 43% of patients [62, 63]. Diagnostic delay of greater than 24 hours occurs in up to 39% of cases [64]. While advanced imaging techniques can reliably diagnose these conditions, it is inefficient, uneconomic and unrealistic to image every patient complaining of chest pain. For the patient with known coronary atherosclerosis, a misdiagnosis of AAD as ACS can have disastrous iatrogenic consequences should the patient receive anticoagulants or thrombolytic therapy [65].

Acute Aortic Dissection: History and Physical Examination

Classically, the pain of AAD is described as sudden onset of severe tearing or ripping chest pain that radiates to the lower back or interscapular region. A meta-analysis of 16 studies and 1553 patients reported that absence of a history of sudden onset chest pain substantially decreases the probability of AAD (LR 0.3). However the presence of this symptom was not diagnostic (LR 1.6) [66]. In addition to chest pain, patients with AAD may present with dyspnea, syncope, neurological deficits and anuria. Other rare clinical presentations include pulsatile sternoclavicular joint, hoarsness, dysphagia, superior vena cava syndrome, Horner's syndrome, bulbar palsies, acute arterial occlusion, deep venous thrombosis and bilateral testicular tenderness [67-71]. Neurological deficits are seen in 17% of patients with AAD. The presence of a neurological deficit with chest pain increases the diagnostic probability (LR 6.6-33.0). However, the absence of this sign does not alter the diagnostic probability.

In cases of suspected AAD, the physical examination focuses on assessment of hemodynamic stability. Blood pressure should be taken in all 4 extremities. Carotid, radial and femoral arteries should be palpated to detect a pulse differential. Cardiac auscultation focuses on detecting a new diastolic murmur of aortic regurgitation. A rapid neurological examination directed towards the detection of gross motor and sensory defects such as hemiplegia and paraplegia should ensue.

A blood pressure difference of 20 mm Hg is considered to be an independent predictor of dissection [61]. The presence of a pulse deficit increases the diagnostic probability (LR 5.7) while absence of this sign does not alter the diagnostic probability for AAD. A meta-analysis found the presence or absence of a diastolic murmur is not helpful as a diagnostic aid [66].

Acute Aortic Dissection: Investigations

Chest radiographic have limited utility for the diagnosis of AAD. Findings that suggest AAD are an abnormal aortic contour, wide mediastinum, new pleural effusions and displaced intimal calcification. Collectively, 90% of patients with AAD have some abnormal finding on a chest radiograph. A completely normal chest radiograph lowers the likelihood of AAD but does not rule it out completely (LR 0.3)[66]. EKG`s also are of limited utility for the diagnosis of AAD. EKG findings of an acute MI do not rule out concomitant AAD.

An inexpensive, widely available and sensitive blood test that physicians can use for an early accurate diagnosis of AAD remains elusive. A D-dimer cutoff level of 500 ng/ml has been shown to have a negative likelihood ratio of 0.007 in patients presenting with chest pain within 24 hours [72]. However, IMH may not show elevation of D dimer and elevated levels may occur in patients with chronic dissection but unrelated chest pain. Further study is needed. Other potential biomarkers for early diagnosis of AAD are the circulating troponin-like proteins of smooth muscle calponin, smooth muscle myosin heavy chain and soluble elastin fragments [73-75].

The main goals in diagnostic imaging are to rapidly confirm (or exclude) an AAD classify the type/extent, assess any side branch involvement, detect acute aortic regurgitation and discover any extravasation into the pericardium, mediastinum and thoracic cavity.

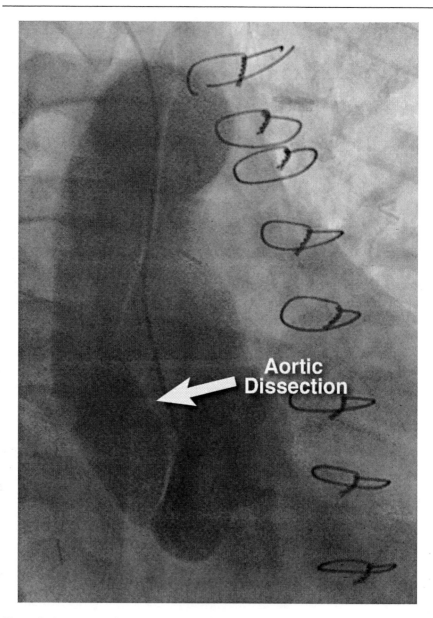

Figure 2. Aortogram of an Acute Aortic Dissection.

A meta-analysis found the sensitivity (98%-100%) and specificity (95%-98%) of magnetic resonance imaging (MRI), helical computed tomography (CT) and transesophageal echocardiography (TEE) to be comparable for confirming or ruling out thoracic aortic dissection [76]. These modalities can also detect other acute aortic syndromes such as IMH and PAU. In suspected AAD early diagnosis is preferred. Therefore, based on a history and physical examination, rapid rule out by the fastest available imaging modality should be the next step. The choice of an imaging modality depends on patient characteristics and local expertise. MRI had the highest value for confirming aortic dissection. Although accurate, this modality is limited by lack of availability, time delay, incompatibility with implanted metal devices and monitoring difficulties during examination. MRI is not suitable for hemodynamically unstable patients. Helical CT is the most widely used modality and had the highest value for ruling out AAD [77]. This is less operator dependant. The disadvantages are need for contrast administration and ionizing radiation. Transthoracic echocardiography has a limited role in diagnosis of AAD, primarily because of its inadequacy in visualizing the distal ascending, transverse and descending aorta. It can identify complications of AAD such as pericardial effusion, aortic regurgitation and assess left ventricular function. TEE is often used with time constraints and in hemodynamically unstable patients. This remains an operator and experience dependant modality. In addition, distal part of the ascending aorta and branches of the aortic arch cannot be adequately evaluated [78]. The frequency of invasive aortography for diagnosis of AAD has decreased 79 as this has a high specificity (94%) but a low sensitivity (88%) for diagnosis (Figure 2) [80 81].

Conclusion

This chapter contains details regarding diagnostic approach to three life threatening diagnoses in a patient with history of coronary atherosclerosis presenting with chest pain.

Key Points

1. Ensuring hemodynamic stability during diagnostic evaluation of patients presenting with chest pain is key.
2. Sudden worsening of ischemic symptoms in a cardiac patient with previously controlled angina and known coronary anatomy should prompt work-up of etiologies for worsening symptoms in addition to investigations to assess plaque rupture.
3. Cardiac biomarker elevation needs to be interpreted within the clinical context and should be remembered as being one of the tools for assessment and management of patients with chest pain.

4. Physical examination in cases of suspected pericarditis is directed to verify the diagnosis and identify presence of pulsus paradoxus.
5. If significant mitral flow velocity respiratory flow variation is present without echocardiographic criteria for moderate or a large pericardial effusion, it is appropriate to perform transesophageal echocardiography to rule out a loculated effusion causing cardiac tamponade in the appropriate clinical scenario.
6. The presence of a neurological deficit a patient presenting with sudden onset of severe tearing or ripping chest pain increases the diagnostic probability of AAD.
7. In patients with suspected AAD a rapid rule out by the fastest available imaging modality (TEE/CT/MRI) should be the next step.

References

[1]   Pope JH, Aufderheide TP, Ruthazer R, et al. Missed diagnoses of acute cardiac ischemia in the emergency department. *N Engl J Med.* Apr 20 2000;342(16):1163-1170.
[2]   Jaffery Z, Hudson MP, Khanal S, et al. The recognition of acute coronary ischemia in the outpatient setting. *J Thromb Thrombolysis.* Jan 2009;27(1):18-23.
[3]   Heberden N. Some account of a disorder of the breast. *Med Transactions* 1772;2:59-67.
[4]   Nawar EW, Niska RW, Xu J. National Hospital Ambulatory Medical Care Survey: 2005 emergency department summary. *Adv Data.* Jun 29 2007(386):1-32.
[5]   Bassan R, Scofano M, Gamarski R, et al. Chest pain in the emergency room. Importance of a systematic approach. *Arq Bras Cardiol.* Jan 2000;74(1):13-29.
[6]   Sonel A, Sasseen BM, Fineberg N, et al. Prospective study correlating fibrinopeptide A, troponin I, myoglobin, and myosin light chain levels with early and late ischemic events in consecutive patients presenting to the emergency department with chest pain. *Circulation.* Sep 5 2000;102(10):1107-1113.
[7]   Hofgren C, Karlson BW, Herlitz J. Prodromal symptoms in subsets of patients hospitalized for suspected acute myocardial infarction. *Heart Lung.* Jan-Feb 1995;24(1):3-10.

[8]   Curtis JP, Schreiner G, Wang Y, et al. All-cause readmission and repeat revascularization after percutaneous coronary intervention in a cohort of medicare patients. *J Am Coll Cardiol.* Sep 1 2009;54(10):903-907.

[9]   Brandrup-Wognsen G, Berggren H, Caidahl K, et al. Predictors for recurrent chest pain and relationship to myocardial ischaemia during long-term follow-up after coronary artery bypass grafting. *Eur J Cardiothorac Surg.* Aug 1997;12(2):304-311.

[10] Lloyd-Jones D, Adams R, Carnethon M, et al. Heart disease and stroke statistics--2009 update: a report from the American Heart Association Statistics Committee and Stroke Statistics Subcommittee. *Circulation.* Jan 27 2009;119(3):480-486.

[11] Lee TH, Rouan GW, Weisberg MC, et al. Clinical characteristics and natural history of patients with acute myocardial infarction sent home from the emergency room. *Am J Cardiol.* Aug 1 1987;60(4):219-224.

[12] Panju AA, Hemmelgarn BR, Guyatt GH, et al. The rational clinical examination. Is this patient having a myocardial infarction? *Jama.* Oct 14 1998;280(14):1256-1263.

[13] Hickam DH, Sox HC, Jr., Sox CH. Systematic bias in recording the history in patients with chest pain. *J Chronic Dis.* 1985;38(1):91-100.

[14] Swap CJ, Nagurney JT. Value and limitations of chest pain history in the evaluation of patients with suspected acute coronary syndromes. *Jama.* Nov 23 2005;294(20):2623-2629.

[15] Constant J. The diagnosis of nonanginal chest pain. *Keio J Med.* Sep 1990;39(3):187-192.

[16] Henrikson CA, Howell EE, Bush DE, et al. Chest pain relief by nitroglycerin does not predict active coronary artery disease. *Ann Intern Med.* Dec 16 2003;139(12):979-986.

[17] Diercks DB, Boghos E, Guzman H, et al. Changes in the numeric descriptive scale for pain after sublingual nitroglycerin do not predict cardiac etiology of chest pain. *Ann Emerg Med.* Jun 2005;45(6):581-585.

[18] Thygesen K, Alpert JS, White HD. Universal definition of myocardial infarction. *J Am Coll Cardiol.* Nov 27 2007;50(22):2173-2195.

[19] Hamm CW. Cardiac biomarkers for rapid evaluation of chest pain. *Circulation.* Sep 25 2001;104(13):1454-1456.

[20] de Winter RJ, Koster RW, Sturk A, et al. Value of myoglobin, troponin T, and CK-MBmass in ruling out an acute myocardial infarction in the emergency room. *Circulation.* Dec 15 1995;92(12):3401-3407.

[21] Morrow DA, Cannon CP, Jesse RL, et al. National Academy of Clinical Biochemistry Laboratory Medicine Practice Guidelines: Clinical

characteristics and utilization of biochemical markers in acute coronary syndromes. *Circulation.* Apr 3 2007;115(13):e356-375.

[22] Guest TM, Ramanathan AV, Tuteur PG, et al. Myocardial injury in critically ill patients. A frequently unrecognized complication. *Jama.* Jun 28 1995;273(24):1945-1949.

[23] Newby LK, Storrow AB, Gibler WB, et al. Bedside multimarker testing for risk stratification in chest pain units: The chest pain evaluation by creatine kinase-MB, myoglobin, and troponin I (CHECKMATE) study. *Circulation.* Apr 10 2001;103(14):1832-1837.

[24] McCann CJ, Glover BM, Menown IB, et al. Investigation of a multimarker approach to the initial assessment of patients with acute chest pain. *Adv Ther.* May 2009;26(5):531-534.

[25] McCann CJ, Glover BM, Menown IB, et al. Novel biomarkers in early diagnosis of acute myocardial infarction compared with cardiac troponin T. *Eur Heart J.* Dec 2008;29(23):2843-2850.

[26] Diamond GA, Forrester JS. Analysis of probability as an aid in the clinical diagnosis of coronary-artery disease. *N Engl J Med.* Jun 14 1979;300(24):1350-1358.

[27] Ishida M, Kato S, Sakuma H. Cardiac MRI in ischemic heart disease. *Circ J.* Sep 2009;73(9):1577-1588.

[28] Lalonde L, Ziadi MC, Beanlands R. Cardiac positron emission tomography: current clinical practice. *Cardiol Clin.* May 2009;27(2):237-255, Table of Contents.

[29] Nandalur KR, Dwamena BA, Choudhri AF, et al. Diagnostic performance of stress cardiac magnetic resonance imaging in the detection of coronary artery disease: a meta-analysis. *J Am Coll Cardiol.* Oct 2 2007;50(14):1343-1353.

[30] Launbjerg J, Fruergaard P, Hesse B, et al. Long-term risk of death, cardiac events and recurrent chest pain in patients with acute chest pain of different origin. *Cardiology.* Jan-Feb 1996;87(1):60-66.

[31] Oliva PB, Hammill SC, Edwards WD. The electrocardiographic diagnosis of regional pericarditis in acute inferior myocardial infarction. *Eur Heart J.* Dec 1993;14(12):1683-1691.

[32] Correale E, Maggioni AP, Romano S, et al. Comparison of frequency, diagnostic and prognostic significance of pericardial involvement in acute myocardial infarction treated with and without thrombolytics. Gruppo Italiano per lo Studio della Sopravvivenza nell'Infarto Miocardico (GISSI). *Am J Cardiol.* Jun 15 1993;71(16):1377-1381.

[33] Correale E, Maggioni AP, Romano S, et al. Pericardial involvement in acute myocardial infarction in the post-thrombolytic era: clinical meaning and value. *Clin Cardiol.* Apr 1997;20(4):327-331.

[34] Aydinalp A, Wishniak A, van den Akker-Berman L, et al. Pericarditis and pericardial effusion in acute ST-elevation myocardial infarction in the thrombolytic era. *Isr Med Assoc J.* Mar 2002;4(3):181-183.

[35] Wall TC, Califf RM, Harrelson-Woodlief L, et al. Usefulness of a pericardial friction rub after thrombolytic therapy during acute myocardial infarction in predicting amount of myocardial damage. The TAMI Study Group. *Am J Cardiol.* Dec 15 1990;66(20):1418-1421.

[36] Cevik C, Wilborn T, Corona R, et al. Post-cardiac injury syndrome following transvenous pacemaker insertion: A case report and review of the literature. *Heart Lung Circ.* Dec 2009;18(6):379-383.

[37] Ito T, Engle MA, Goldberg HP. Postpericardiotomy syndrome following surgery for nonrheumatic heart disease. *Circulation.* Apr 1958;17(4, Part 1):549-556.

[38] Dressler W, Leavitt SS. Pericarditis after acute myocardial infarction. Relapses over period of twenty-eight months. *Jama.* Jul 16 1960;173:1225-1226.

[39] Greene TO, Portnow AS, Huang SK. Acute pericarditis resulting from an endocardial active fixation screw-in atrial lead. *Pacing Clin Electrophysiol.* Jan 1994;17(1):21-25.

[40] Mahapatra S, Bybee KA, Bunch TJ, et al. Incidence and predictors of cardiac perforation after permanent pacemaker placement. *Heart Rhythm.* Sep 2005;2(9):907-911.

[41] Fasseas P, Orford JL, Panetta CJ, et al. Incidence, correlates, management, and clinical outcome of coronary perforation: analysis of 16,298 procedures. *Am Heart J.* Jan 2004;147(1):140-145.

[42] Javaid A, Buch AN, Satler LF, et al. Management and outcomes of coronary artery perforation during percutaneous coronary intervention. *Am J Cardiol.* Oct 1 2006;98(7):911-914.

[43] Lange RA, Hillis LD. Clinical practice. Acute pericarditis. *N Engl J Med.* Nov 18 2004;351(21):2195-2202.

[44] Roy CL, Minor MA, Brookhart MA, et al. Does this patient with a pericardial effusion have cardiac tamponade? *Jama.* Apr 25 2007;297(16):1810-1818.

[45] Zayas R, Anguita M, Torres F, et al. Incidence of specific etiology and role of methods for specific etiologic diagnosis of primary acute pericarditis. *Am J Cardiol.* Feb 15 1995;75(5):378-382.

[46] Spodick DH. Pericardial rub. Prospective, Multiple observer investigation of pericardial friction in 100 patients. *Am J Cardiol.* Mar 1975;35(3):357-362.

[47] Spodick DH. Diagnostic electrocardiographic sequences in acute pericarditis. Significance of PR segment and PR vector changes. *Circulation.* Sep 1973;48(3):575-580.

[48] Oliva PB, Hammill SC, Edwards WD. Electrocardiographic diagnosis of postinfarction regional pericarditis. Ancillary observations regarding the effect of reperfusion on the rapidity and amplitude of T wave inversion after acute myocardial infarction. *Circulation.* Sep 1993;88(3):896-904.

[49] Sugiura T, Iwasaka T, Takayama Y, et al. Factors associated with pericardial effusion in acute Q wave myocardial infarction. *Circulation.* Feb 1990;81(2):477-481.

[50] Widimsky P, Gregor P. Pericardial involvement during the course of myocardial infarction. A long-term clinical and echocardiographic study. *Chest.* Jul 1995;108(1):89-93.

[51] Dorfman TA, Aqel R. Regional pericarditis: a review of the pericardial manifestations of acute myocardial infarction. *Clin Cardiol.* Mar 2009;32(3):115-120.

[52] Troughton RW, Asher CR, Klein AL. Pericarditis. *Lancet.* Feb 28 2004;363(9410):717-727.

[53] Maisch B, Seferovic PM, Ristic AD, et al. Guidelines on the diagnosis and management of pericardial diseases executive summary; The Task force on the diagnosis and management of pericardial diseases of the European society of cardiology. *Eur Heart J.* Apr 2004;25(7):587-610.

[54] Saito Y, Donohue A, Attai S, et al. The syndrome of cardiac tamponade with "small" pericardial effusion. *Echocardiography.* Mar 2008;25(3):321-327.

[55] Sarasin FP, Louis-Simonet M, Gaspoz JM, et al. Detecting acute thoracic aortic dissection in the emergency department: time constraints and choice of the optimal diagnostic test. *Ann Emerg Med.* Sep 1996;28(3):278-288.

[56] Erbel R, Alfonso F, Boileau C, et al. Diagnosis and management of aortic dissection. *Eur Heart J.* Sep 2001;22(18):1642-1681.

[57] Evangelista A, Mukherjee D, Mehta RH, et al. Acute intramural hematoma of the aorta: a mystery in evolution. *Circulation.* Mar 1 2005;111(8):1063-1070.

[58] Moizumi Y, Komatsu T, Motoyoshi N, et al. Management of patients with intramural hematoma involving the ascending aorta. *J Thorac Cardiovasc Surg.* Nov 2002;124(5):918-924.

[59] Motoyoshi N, Moizumi Y, Komatsu T, et al. Intramural hematoma and dissection involving ascending aorta: the clinical features and prognosis. *Eur J Cardiothorac Surg.* Aug 2003;24(2):237-242; discussion 242.

[60] Song JK, Yim JH, Ahn JM, et al. Outcomes of patients with acute type a aortic intramural hematoma. *Circulation.* Nov 24 2009;120(21):2046-2052.

[61] von Kodolitsch Y, Schwartz AG, Nienaber CA. Clinical prediction of acute aortic dissection. *Arch Intern Med.* Oct 23 2000;160(19):2977-2982.

[62] Sullivan PR, Wolfson AB, Leckey RD, et al. Diagnosis of acute thoracic aortic dissection in the emergency department. *Am J Emerg Med.* Jan 2000;18(1):46-50.

[63] Meszaros I, Morocz J, Szlavi J, et al. Epidemiology and clinicopathology of aortic dissection. *Chest.* May 2000;117(5):1271-1278.

[64] Viljanen T. Diagnostic difficulties in aortic dissection. Retrospective study of 89 surgically treated patients. *Ann Chir Gynaecol.* 1986;75(6):328-332.

[65] Marian AJ, Harris SL, Pickett JD, et al. Inadvertent administration of rtPA to a patient with type 1 aortic dissection and subsequent cardiac tamponade. *Am J Emerg Med.* Nov 1993;11(6):613-615.

[66] Klompas M. Does this patient have an acute thoracic aortic dissection? *Jama.* May 1 2002;287(17):2262-2272.

[67] Chan-Tack KM. Aortic dissection presenting as bilateral testicular pain. *N Engl J Med.* Oct 19 2000;343(16):1199.

[68] Eagle KA, Quertermous T, Kritzer GA, et al. Spectrum of conditions initially suggesting acute aortic dissection but with negative aortograms. *Am J Cardiol.* Feb 1 1986;57(4):322-326.

[69] Gleeson H, Hughes T, Northridge D, et al. Bulbar palsies and chest pain. *Lancet.* Sep 2 2000;356(9232):826.

[70] Robertson GS, Macpherson DS. Aortic aneurysm presenting as deep venous thrombosis. *Lancet.* Apr 16 1988;1(8590):877-878.

[71] Pacifico L, Spodick D. ILEAD--ischemia of the lower extremities due to aortic dissection: the isolated presentation. *Clin Cardiol.* May 1999;22(5):353-356.

[72] Suzuki T, Distante A, Zizza A, et al. Diagnosis of acute aortic dissection by D-dimer: the International Registry of Acute Aortic Dissection Substudy on Biomarkers (IRAD-Bio) experience. *Circulation.* May 26 2009;119(20):2702-2707.

[73] Suzuki T, Distante A, Zizza A, et al. Preliminary experience with the smooth muscle troponin-like protein, calponin, as a novel biomarker for diagnosing acute aortic dissection. *Eur Heart J.* Jun 2008;29(11):1439-1445.

[74] Suzuki T, Katoh H, Tsuchio Y, et al. Diagnostic implications of elevated levels of smooth-muscle myosin heavy-chain protein in acute aortic dissection. The smooth muscle myosin heavy chain study. *Ann Intern Med.* Oct 3 2000; 133(7):537-541.

[75] Shinohara T, Suzuki K, Okada M, et al. Soluble elastin fragments in serum are elevated in acute aortic dissection. *Arterioscler Thromb Vasc Biol.* Oct 1 2003; 23(10):1839-1844.

[76] Shiga T, Wajima Z, Apfel CC, et al. Diagnostic accuracy of transesophageal echocardiography, helical computed tomography, and magnetic resonance imaging for suspected thoracic aortic dissection: systematic review and meta-analysis. *Arch Intern Med.* Jul 10 2006;166(13): 1350-1356.

[77] Hagan PG, Nienaber CA, Isselbacher EM, et al. The International Registry of Acute Aortic Dissection (IRAD): new insights into an old disease. *Jama.* Feb 16 2000;283(7):897-903.

[78] Borner N, Erbel R, Braun B, et al. Diagnosis of aortic dissection by transesophageal echocardiography. *Am J Cardiol.* Nov 1 1984; 54(8):1157-1158.

[79] Cigarroa JE, Isselbacher EM, DeSanctis RW, et al. Diagnostic imaging in the evaluation of suspected aortic dissection. Old standards and new directions. *N Engl J Med.* Jan 7 1993;328(1):35-43.

[80] Dinsmore RE, Rourke JA, DeSanctis RD, et al. Angiographic findings in dissecting aortic aneurysm. *N Engl J Med.* Nov 24 1966;275(21):1152-1157.

[81] Erbel R, Engberding R, Daniel W, et al. Echocardiography in diagnosis of aortic dissection. *Lancet.* Mar 4 1989;1(8636):457-461.

In: Chest Pain Causes, Diagnosis and Treatment   ISBN 978-1-61728-112-9
Editor: Sophie M. Weber, pp. 119-133   © 2010 Nova Science Publishers, Inc.

Chapter 5

Chest Pain: Angina

M. Justin S. Zaman [*] *and Phyo Kyaw Myint*[†]

[1].University College London, London, UK
[2]. School of Medicine, Health Policy and Practice,
University of East Anglia,
Norwich, NR4 7TJ, UK

Abstract

Angina is one of the commonest causes of chest pain. It is a common initial manifestation of coronary heart disease, a significant burden in primary care and has considerable economic implications globally. Angina is usually diagnosed from a clinical constellation of symptoms from the patient's history. Descriptions of symptoms, articulated by patients to their doctors, remain a cornerstone of diagnosis in clinical medicine. Whilst the diagnosis of angina is straight forward in many cases, it can be difficult in certain circumstances such as older people and people presenting with atypical symptoms. There have been recent developments in European guidelines for the diagnosis of angina. In this chapter we will describe the definition, causes of angina and its differential diagnosis. We will also discuss its management from primary and secondary prevention and treatment perspectives.

[*] Tel: + 44 (0) 20 3108 3082, Fax: +44 (0) 20 7813 0242, Mail to: j.zaman@ucl.ac.uk.
[†] Tel: + 44 (0) 1603 286286. Fax: +44 (0) 1603 286428.Mail to: phyo.k.myint@uea.ac.uk.

Introduction

Angina is a common initial manifestation of coronary heart disease,[1] a significant burden in primary care[2] and has considerable economic implications. A UK study conservatively estimated that angina accounted for 1.3% of the annual health expenditure.[3]

Definition

Angina is diagnosed from a clinical constellation of symptoms from the patient history. Descriptions of symptoms, articulated by patients to their doctors, remain a cornerstone of diagnosis in clinical medicine. The clinical history is the first step in assessing chest pain or discomfort in order to ascertain whether or not it represents angina. The history also allows the doctor to identify patients in whom additional investigation is necessary and in whom it may be spared,[4 5] and whether additional therapy including coronary revascularisation through percutaneous coronary intervention (PCI, using balloon angioplasty and stenting) or coronary artery bypass surgery (CABG) is needed.

Diamond and Forrester Definition

One of the most widely used definitions of chronic stable angina pectoris was presented in 1979 by Diamond and Forrester who analysed 4952 patients with chest discomfort. They showed that typicality of symptoms correlated with angiographic coronary disease.[5] The authors described three types of chest pain: nonanginal, atypical, and typical.

The pain was assessed with these questions:

1) Is the pain retrosternal?
2) Is the pain precipitated by stress?
3) Is the pain relieved by rest or nitroglycerin?

Patients who answer yes to all three questions were determined to have typical chest pain, those who answered yes to two of the questions to have atypical chest pain and those who answered yes to only one question were deemed to have nonanginal chest pain.

European Task Force Definition

The Task Force on the Management of Stable Angina Pectoris of the European Society of Cardiology defined angina as follows in its 2006 consensus document:[6]

"Stable angina is a clinical syndrome characterized by discomfort in the chest, jaw, shoulder, back, or arms, typically elicited by exertion or emotional stress and relieved by rest or nitroglycerin".

It continued:

"The characteristics of discomfort related to myocardial ischaemia (angina pectoris) have been extensively described and may be divided into four types: location, character, duration and relation to exertion, and other exacerbating or relieving factors. The discomfort caused by myocardial ischaemia is usually located in the chest, near the sternum, but may be felt anywhere from the epigastrium to the lower jaw or teeth, between the shoulder blades or in either arm to the wrist and fingers. The discomfort is usually described as pressure, tightness, or heaviness, sometimes strangling, constricting, or burning. The severity of the discomfort varies greatly and is not related to the severity of the underlying coronary disease. Shortness of breath may accompany angina, and chest discomfort may also be accompanied by less specific symptoms such as fatigue or faintness, nausea, burping, restlessness, or a sense of impending dooms".

The duration of the discomfort is brief, not more than 10 minutes in the majority of cases, and more commonly even less. An important characteristic is the relation to exercise, specific activities, or emotional stress. Symptoms classically deteriorate with increased levels of exertion, such as walking up an incline or against a breeze, and rapidly disappear within a few minutes, when these causal factors abate. Exacerbations of symptoms after a heavy meal or first thing in the morning are classical features of angina. Buccal or sublingual nitrates rapidly relieve angina, and a similar rapid response may be observed with chewing nifedipine capsules".

Finally, to classify, it presented the following classification:
Typical angina (definite)- Meets three of the following characteristics

- Substernal chest discomfort of characteristic quality and duration
- Provoked by exertion or emotional stress
- Relieved by rest and/or GTN (glyceryl trinitrate)

Atypical angina (probable)- Meets two of the above characteristics
Non-cardiac chest pain - Meets one or none of the above

This definition outlined what constitutes typical characteristics of angina pectoris, and framed it into the categories of location, character, duration and relation to exertion, and other exacerbating or relieving factors. What constitutes typical characteristics of angina was not specified in the Diamond and Forrester definition.

The Rose Angina Questionnaire

The Rose angina questionnaire (RQ) is a widely-used survey tool for the measuring of angina in populations.[7] The questionnaire was introduced in 1962 and defines angina as chest pain that limits exertion, is situated over the sternum or in the left chest and left arm, and is relieved within 10 minutes by rest. It is highly specific when compared against a medical record of doctor-diagnosed angina,[8] and is strongly associated with subsequent risk of coronary events in European populations.[9] This definition outlines typical characteristics of angina pectoris within the categories of location, duration and relation to exertion.

Measuring Angina

The early and appropriate identification of angina will result in early and appropriate investigation and treatment.[4 5]

Typicality of Angina

While laboratories standardise assays for biomarkers in the measurement of a myocardial infarction, angina is a clinical constellation of symptom descriptors, rendering quantitative measurement difficult. There are few large studies comparing the diagnostic and prognostic value of chest pain descriptors between different populations, as symptoms have been predominately investigated in White male populations. The difficulty in measuring angina as a phenotype was highlighted in a 2001 cross-sectional study where the reliability of the Rose angina questionnaire was reported to be inconsistent in South Asian populations when compared to self-reported doctor-diagnosed angina and independently coded electrocardiogram (ECG) abnormalities.[10] The Rose Angina Questionnaire has been used as a cardiovascular disease health indicator for decades and is still in widespread use in epidemiological studies. However, the Rose Angina Questionnaire was developed as a screening tool in Western countries when coronary heart disease incidence and mortality was far higher than today. More discriminating measurement of angina symptoms, focusing more on the description and consistency of the chest pain, may complement existing angina assessment. Using a multi-centre chest pain clinic cohort, descriptors of chest pain using a simple symptom score were predictive of coronary events across sex and ethnicity.[11] However, significant numbers of patients with atypical histories remained at risk of future coronary events.

Severity of Angina

Ambulatory patients reporting a significant deterioration in their angina over the preceding month have been found to have a higher one-year mortality rate than those with more stable symptoms.[12] Furthermore, a higher burden of symptoms is associated with higher physical and role functioning.[13] As angina has potentially adverse prognoses both in terms of mortality and morbidity if not adequately managed, accurate measurement of its severity is of clinical importance.

The Canadian Cardiovascular Society (CCS) classification system has been used as an epidemiological tool to measure the severity of angina.[14] Worse severity of angina on the CCS score is associated with a more adverse prognosis as measured by rates of myocardial infarction and death.[15] This measure is a scale ranging from I, when angina is mild and does not limit physical activity, through to IV, when angina severely restricts activities (box below).

Table I. Canadian Cardiovascular Society Functional Classification of Angina

Class	Activity Evoking Angina	Limits to Physical Activity
I	Prolonged exertion	None
II	Walking > 2 blocks or > 1 flight of stairs	Slight
III	Walking < 2 blocks or < 1 flight of stairs	Marked
IV	Minimal or at rest	Severe

Prevalence of Angina

Around two million women and men in the UK have angina and about 1% of the population visit their general practitioner at least once yearly with symptoms of angina.[16] National surveys have produced data on the prevalence of angina in the UK, as tabulated below (Table II). In a meta-analysis on the international prevalence of angina, angina varied from 0.73% to 14.4% in women (population weighted mean, 6.7%) and 0.76% to 15.1% in men (population weighted mean, 5.7%).[1]

The incidence of diagnosed angina appears to be increasing when examining secular trends from 1978 to 2000. This is in contrast to a decline in rates of all other types of major coronary events among British men.[17] General practice morbidity survey data from England and Wales also indicates that angina may be increasing,[2] with the rate of consultation for angina among men and women in the 1990s higher than in the 1980s, the comparable statistic for myocardial infarction having fallen during this time. Contrasting evidence from the British Regional Heart Study reported that the prevalence of angina symptoms fell from 1978-1996, among men with and without a diagnosis of coronary heart disease.[18]This was a study in which angina was defined in a standardised way throughout follow-up.

Table II. Prevalence of angina in UK adults from survey data

Study, year	Study population	Definition of angina	Prevalence of angina (%)			
			Ages 55-64		Ages 65-74	
			Women	Men	Women	Men
Health survey for England, 2006*	Random sample of addresses - 14,142 adults interviewed	Rose Angina Questionnaire/Self-reported doctor-diagnosed angina	3.3/3.2	3.6/8.0	5.0/8.3	4.9/14.2
The Scottish Health Survey, 2003**	Random sample of addresses - 8,148 adults interviewed	Rose Angina Questionnaire/Self-reported doctor-diagnosed angina	4.0/7.4	5.1/11.2	16.8/14.2	6.7/20.8

* http://www.ic.nhs.uk/statistics
**http://www.scotland.gov.uk/Publications/2005/11/25145024/50253

However, this reported finding is limited by the authors' technique of determining overall population prevalence of angina through the use of a series of cross sectional studies nested within what is a prospective cohort study.

Though analyses were age-adjusted, the presented 'trend' in prevalence of angina should be interpreted cautiously. Their findings of a decline in age-specific angina prevalence are more robust among the men aged between 55 and 64 years, who contributed to at least three of the cross sectional studies. Data from successive Health Surveys for England can provide information on such trends and overall show no evidence of any significant change in the prevalence of self reported symptoms as assessed by the Rose Questionnaire between 1991 and 1994 and only a small, non-significant decline in men between 1994 and 1998.[19] Thus, a valid measurement of chest pain is important for the true assessment of prevalence.

Treatment of Angina

The management of angina comprises two main strategies:

- Anti-anginal medication - β-blockers, calcium-channel antagonists, nitrates and potassium-channel activators like nicorandil
- Coronary revascularisation (following investigation by invasive coronary angiography) – percutaneously by balloon angioplasty/ stenting, or surgically through bypass grafting.

Many patients with angina are not investigated through coronary angiography, as symptoms may settle on medication alone. As the risk of death from coronary angiography is around 1 in 1000,[20] the purpose of coronary angiography is to plan a management strategy beyond medication alone that will improve the patient's quality of life or prognosis. American College of Cardiology/American Heart Association Guidelines for Coronary Angiography[21] recommend invasive investigation in patients with CCS class III and IV angina despite being on anti-anginal medication.

Prognosis of Angina

In patients with a diagnosis of angina, it has been reported that 17% will have died from coronary heart disease or been admitted with a non-fatal myocardial infarction or unstable angina within three years.[1]

Prognosis of angina can be investigated both in terms of:

- the future risk of serious manifestations of coronary disease such as unstable angina, myocardial infarction and coronary death;
- as an outcome itself, as those who suffer angina and undergo treatment to allay their symptoms may have their symptoms return (symptomatic prognosis).

Risk of Future Myocardial Infarction and Coronary Death

In those patients with exertional angina, prognosis for myocardial infarction and death is not improved by coronary revascularisation:

- A meta-analysis of randomised controlled trials in 2000 comparing PTCA (percutaneous trans-luminal coronary angioplasty, balloon angioplasty alone without stenting) with medical treatment alone in chronic coronary heart disease concluded that PTCA led to a reduction in angina (relative risk (RR) 0.70 (95% confidence interval (CI) 0.50-0.98)) but conferred no beneficial effects on risk of myocardial infarction or death.[22]
- In the Second Randomized Intervention Treatment of Angina (RITA-2),[23] death or myocardial infarction occurred in 73 (14.5%) PTCA patients and 63 (12.3%) medical patients (p=0.21).
- A 1994 meta-analysis compared CABG with medical treatment and found that surgery conferred a survival advantage only in those patients with severe left main stem coronary disease, three-vessel disease, or two-vessel disease with a severely stenosed proximal left anterior descending artery.[24] However, only 10% of trial patients received an internal mammary artery graft in addition to their vein grafts, routine practice in current surgery now. Only 25% received anti-platelet drugs whilst use of statins was similarly low compared to current standards.

Secondary prevention medical therapy (aspirin, statins) on the other hand plays a role in the stabilisation of the atherosclerotic process, as shown in studies such as the REVERSAL study, where intensive lipid-lowering treatment with statins reduced the progression of coronary atherosclerosis as measured by intravascular ultrasound.[25] The effect of cholesterol lowering with statins on mortality and morbidity in patients with coronary heart disease is well-known, first muted on a large scale by the 4S study,[26] and subsequently shown on meta-analysis of 4S and four subsequent trials.[27]

Risk of Future Recurrent Angina

The importance of revascularisation in improving symptomatic outcomes has been shown in both meta-analyses[22] and large clinical trials.[12] However, studies have documented that many patients undergoing revascularisation still have angina after one year.[28 29] Few studies examine morbidity in the form of symptomatic outcomes following revascularisation yet coronary revascularisation for angina is performed primarily for relief of symptoms. Assessing prognosis for 'hard' outcomes such as myocardial infarction and death is of equal importance to studying symptomatic prognosis.

Differential Diagnosis Of Angina

The following diagnoses of chest pain should be considered when diagnosing angina-
Chest wall – musculosleletal chest pain/costochondral pain

- Palpation tenderness
- Chest pain exacerbated by chest (e.g. twisting the body)

Pulmonary embolism (PE)

- Dyspnoea
- Pleuritic in nature (exacerbated by taking deep breath)
- Associated hypoxia
- Cyanosis and shock in severe cases

Pneumonia

- Dyspnoea
- Pleuritic in nature (exacerbated by taking deep breath)
- Associated hypoxia
- Symptoms of pneumonia (cough, sputum production, fever)
- Spontaneous pneumothorax
- Dyspnoea
- History of bullous emphysema may present

- Typical CXR appearance

Aortic dissection

- Severe pain (may typically present with tearing pain radiate through to back)
- Signs of impending infero-posterior infarction (type A dissection sometimes obstructs the origin of a coronary artery- usually the right)
- Asymmetrical pulses and blood pressure
- New aortic valve regurgitation
- Shock in severe cases
- CXR may show widened mediastinum

Pericarditis

- Pain influenced by changing posture and breathing
- A friction sound (pericardial rub) may be heard on auscultation
- ST elevation but no reciprocal ST depression (generalised ST elevation)

Pleurisy

- Stabbing (sharp) pain with breathing
- May have signs and symptoms of PE or pneumonia

Ectopic beats

- Occur also at rest
- Apical location (at apex)
- Transient

Early herpes zoster

- Localised paraesthesia
- No ECG changes
- Rash appears after a couple of days

Oesophageal spasm and reflux oesophagitis

- Worse in recumbent position
- Heartburn
- No ECG changes

Peptic ulcer, cholecystitis, pancreatitis

- Suggestive history and clinical examination -examination of the abdomen!

Depression

- Heaviness in the chest
- Continuous symptom (no correlation to exercise)
- Signs and symptoms suggestive of depressive illness

Hyperventilation syndrome

- Dyspnoea
- Tingling and numbness of the limbs
- Dizziness
- Low CO_2 level
- May occur secondarily due to an organic illness or cause- e.g. acidosis, PE, acute asthma, pneumothorax

Conclusion

With the increasing ageing populations and westernisation of lifestyle in many developing countries, the magnitude of the problem of coronary heart disease (CHD) is likely to increase in the future. Angina is the common manifestation of the ischaemic heart disease and the recognition and appropriate management is pivotal in reducing global burden of CHD. In this chapter, we review the definition of angina; provide its management and prognosis and differential diagnosis for practicing clinicians to aid better understanding of angina and its management.

References

[1] Sekhri N, Feder GS, Junghans C, Hemingway H, Timmis AD. Rapid-access chest pain clinics and the traditional cardiology out-patient clinic. *QJM* 2006;99(March 1, 2006):135-141.

[2] McCormick A, Fleming, D., Charlton, J. Morbidity statistics from general practice. Fourth national study, 1991-1992. London: HMSO: Royal College of General Practitioners, Office of Population Censuses and Surveys, Department of Health, 1995.

[3] Stewart S, Murphy N, Walker A, McGuire A, McMurray JJV. The current cost of angina pectoris to the National Health Service in the UK. *Heart* 2003;89(8):848-853.

[4] Nease RF, Jr., Kneeland T, O'Connor GT, Sumner W, Lumpkins C, Shaw L, et al. Variation in patient utilities for outcomes of the management of chronic stable angina. Implications for clinical practice guidelines. Ischemic Heart Disease Patient Outcomes Research Team. *Jama* 1995;273(15):1185-90.

[5] Diamond GA. A clinically relevant classification of chest discomfort. *J Am Coll Cardiol* 1983;1(2 Pt 1):574-5.

[6] Sutcliffe SJ, Fox KF, Wood DA, Sutcliffe A, Stock K, Wright M, et al. Incidence of coronary heart disease in a health authority in London: review of a community register. *BMJ* 2003;326(7379):20-.

[7] Rose G, Blackburn, H. Cardiovascular Survey Methods. Geneva: World Health Organization, 1968:527-536.

[8] Lawlor DA, Adamson J, Ebrahim S. Performance of the WHO Rose angina questionnaire in post-menopausal women: Are all of the questions necessary? *J Epidemiol Community Health* 2003;57(July 1, 2003):538-541.

[9] Lampe FC, Whincup PH, Shaper AG, Wannamethee SG, Walker M, Ebrahim S. Variability of angina symptoms and the risk of major ischemic heart disease events. *Am J Epidemiol* 2001;153(12):1173-82.

[10] Fischbacher CM, Bhopal R, Unwin N, White M, Alberti K. The performance of the Rose angina questionnaire in South Asian and European origin populations: a comparative study in Newcastle, UK. *Int. J. Epidemiol.* 2001;30(5):1009-1016.

[11] Zaman MJ, Junghans, C., Sekhri, N., Chen, R., Feder, G., Timmis, A., Hemingway, H. Presentation of stable angina pectoris among women and South Asian people. *CMAJ* 2008;179(7):659-667.

[12] Boden WE, O'Rourke RA, Teo KK, Hartigan PM, Maron DJ, Kostuk WJ, et al. Optimal Medical Therapy with or without PCI for Stable Coronary Disease. *N Engl J Med* 2007(March 26, 2007): NEJMoa070829.

[13] Pocock SJ, Henderson RA, Seed P, Treasure T, Hampton JR. Quality of life, employment status, and anginal symptoms after coronary angioplasty or bypass surgery. 3-year follow-up in the Randomized Intervention Treatment of Angina (RITA) Trial. *Circulation* 1996;94(2):135-42.

[14] Campeau L. Grading of angina pectoris [letter]. *Circulation* 1976; 54:522-523.

[15] Daly CA, De Stavola B, Sendon JL, Tavazzi L, Boersma E, Clemens F, et al. Predicting prognosis in stable angina--results from the Euro heart survey of stable angina: prospective observational study. *Bmj* 2006;332(7536):262-7.

[16] http://www.heartstats.org/homepage.asp: British Heart Foundation Statistics Website, 2005.

[17] Lampe FC, Morris RW, Walker M, Shaper AG, Whincup PH. Trends in rates of different forms of diagnosed coronary heart disease, 1978 to 2000: prospective, population based study of British men. *BMJ* 2005;330(7499):1046-.

[18] Lampe FC, Morris RW, Whincup PH, Walker M, Ebrahim S, Shaper AG. Is the prevalence of coronary heart disease falling in British men? *Heart* 2001;86(5):499-505.

[19] Primatesta P. *Prevalence of cardiovascular disease*. London: The Stationery Office, 1999.

[20] Bernstein S, Laouri, M, Hilbourne, LH, Leape, LL, Kahan, JO, Park, RE, et al. *Coronary angiography: a literature review and ratings of appropriateness and necessity*. Santa Monica, CA: RAND, 1992.

[21] Scanlon PJ, Faxon DP, Audet A-M, Carabello B, Dehmer GJ, Eagle KA, et al. ACC/AHA Guidelines for Coronary Angiography: Executive Summary and Recommendations : A Report of the American College of Cardiology/American Heart Association Task Force on Practice Guidelines (Committee on Coronary Angiography) Developed in collaboration with the Society for Cardiac Angiography and Interventions. *Circulation* 1999;99(17):2345-2357.

[22] Bucher HC, Hengstler P, Schindler C, Guyatt GH. Percutaneous transluminal coronary angioplasty versus medical treatment for non-

acute coronary heart disease: meta-analysis of randomised controlled trials. *BMJ* 2000;321(7253):73-7.

[23] Henderson RA, Pocock SJ, Clayton TC, Knight R, Fox KA, Julian DG, et al. Seven-year outcome in the RITA-2 trial: coronary angioplasty versus medical therapy. *J Am Coll Cardiol* 2003;42(7):1161-70.

[24] Yusuf S, Zucker D, Peduzzi P, Fisher LD, Takaro T, Kennedy JW, et al. Effect of coronary artery bypass graft surgery on survival: overview of 10-year results from randomised trials by the Coronary Artery Bypass Graft Surgery Trialists Collaboration. *Lancet* 1994;344(8922):563-70.

[25] Nissen SE, Tuzcu EM, Schoenhagen P, Crowe T, Sasiela WJ, Tsai J, et al. Statin Therapy, LDL Cholesterol, C-Reactive Protein, and Coronary Artery Disease. *N Engl J Med* 2005;352(January 6, 2005):29-38.

[26] Randomised trial of cholesterol lowering in 4444 patients with coronary heart disease: the Scandinavian Simvastatin Survival Study (4S). *Lancet* 1994;344(8934):1383-9.

[27] LaRosa JC, He J, Vupputuri S. Effect of Statins on Risk of Coronary Disease: A Meta-analysis of Randomized Controlled Trials. *JAMA* 1999;282(December 22, 1999):2340-2346.

[28] Serruys PW, Unger F, Sousa JE, Jatene A, Bonnier HJRM, Schonberger JPAM, et al. Comparison of Coronary-Artery Bypass Surgery and Stenting for the Treatment of Multivessel Disease. *N Engl J Med* 2001;344(15):1117-1124.

[29] Poole-Wilson PA, Voko Z, Kirwan BA, de Brouwer S, Dunselman PH, Lubsen J. Clinical course of isolated stable angina due to coronary heart disease. *Eur Heart J* 2007;28(16):1928-35.

In: Chest Pain Causes, Diagnosis and Treatment   ISBN 978-1-61728-112-9
Editor: Sophie M. Weber, pp. 135-140   © 2010 Nova Science Publishers, Inc.

Chapter 6

Ambient Nitrogen Dioxide and Female ED Visits for Chest Pain

M. Szyszkowicz [*]
Population Studies Division, Health Canada, Ottawa, Ontario

Abstract

Objectives: Ambient exposure to nitrogen dioxide (NO_2) has been previously associated with the occurrence of chest pain. The objective of the current study was to examine the correlation between ambient nitrogen dioxide concentrations and emergency department (ED) visits for chest pain in Toronto, Canada. *Design and Methods*: This was a case-crossover study of ED visits for chest pain in female patients that were recorded at one hospital. In the constructed conditional logistic regression models, temperature and relative humidity were adjusted in the form of natural splines with 3 degrees of freedom. The calculations were completed for a sequence of 47 overlapping age groups: [20, 39], [21, 40], and so on, up to [66, 85]. The results, expressed as odds ratios (ORs) and their respective 95% confidence intervals (95% CI), were reported for an increase in the interquartile range (IQR = $75^{th} - 25^{th}$ percentiles; IQR = 9.9 ppb). *Results:* The results were summarized in two figures. One figure shows the OR values and their respective 95% CIs; another represents median values and two quartiles (1 and 3) for controls and

---

[*] Author for correspondence: Dr. Mieczyslaw Szyszkowicz, Health Canada, 269 Laurier Avenue, Room 3-030, Ottawa, ON, K1A 0K9, Canada, Phone: (613) 946-3542, Fax: (613) 948-8482, Email: mietek.szyszkowicz@hc-sc.gc.ca.

cases, both for 47 age groups. Positive and statistically significant associations were observed for patients in the age interval [39, 72] years; the OR = 1.10 (95% CI: 1.00, 1.22). *Conclusions:* Our findings provide additional support for an association between NO$_2$ exposure and the number of ED visits for chest pain in female patients.

This study was inspired by recent publications [1-2] on ambient air pollution exposure and emergency department (ED) visits for chest pain. The published results suggested an association between ambient nitrogen dioxide (NO$_2$) exposure and ED visits this condition.

The purpose of this study was to assess the relationship between urban ambient nitrogen dioxide exposure and female ED visits for chest pain in Toronto, Canada. The study was based on time-series data comprising daily summarized ED chest pain visits (daily counts). We constructed models for a single ambient air pollutant and adjusted for temperature and relative humidity. A case-crossover (CC) design [3] was applied in the study.

Materials and Methods

Study Population

The population considered in this study consisted of patients served by a hospital in Toronto, Canada. We considered the period of April 1, 1999 to March 31, 2002, and restricted the study population to patients in the age interval [0, 85] years.

Statistical Methods

The CC technique is an adaptation of the case–control approach [3]. By definition of the case-crossover methodology, the cases served as their own controls on a set of predefined control days proximate to the time they became cases. A time-stratified approach to determine controls was adopted, as it has been demonstrated to produce unbiased conditional logistic regression estimates [4]. In this design, the controls are matched to case periods by day of week for each case period, and the control periods are determined as other days in the same month and year. This strategy was applied here; thus, there are 3 or 4 controls for each case.

The generated results were reported as the odds ratios (ORs) and their corresponding 95% confidence intervals (95% CI). The ORs were reported for an increase in the nitrogen dioxide concentration represented as the interquartile range (IQR = Q3 − Q1 = 75th − 25th values of percentiles, IQR = 9.9 ppb) of concentrations. Temperature and relative humidity were adjusted in the form of natural splines with 3 degrees of freedom. In the constructed models, values of nitrogen dioxide concentrations and meteorological factors were recorded on the same day as the visit (case) day.

The sequence of 47 overlapping age groups, each of length 20 years, was defined in the following way: the first age group was [20, 29], the second [1, 30], and each successive one was created from the current one by shifting it by one year. In this sequence the last element was defined to be the age group [66, 85]. For the age intervals in this sequence the CC analysis was performed separately. The results for the age sequencing are reported only for female patients.

Results

We applied the ICD-9 codes [5] to identify the ED cases classified as chest pain using the 786.X rubric. We obtained data on 6,652 ED visits diagnosed as chest pain, of which 3,378 cases (51%) were females and the focus of this study.

The main results are organized in the form of two summary figures. Figure 1 represents the values of the ORs and their corresponding 95% CIs. Figure 2 shows the nitrogen dioxide exposure levels for controls and cases (the estimated median; first and third quartiles, Q1 and Q3), and also indicates the number of cases (divided by 30) in the considered age group.

Our analysis revealed positive and significant correlations between nitrogen dioxide exposure and female ED visits for chest pain. The results were statistically significant for the patients in the age interval [39 - 72] years; the OR = 1.10 (95% CI: 1.00, 1.22). In cases where the ORs were greater than 1, i.e., the age interval [28 -77], the OR = 0.92 (95% CI: 0.83, 1.04). For all female patients, the OR = 1.02 (95% CI: 0.95, 1.09); for those not older than age 66, the OR = 1.09 (95% CI: 0.99, 1.19); and for the patients older than 65 (i.e., 65+) years, the OR = 0.92 (95% CI: 0.83, 1.04). For male patients the results were not statistically significant; for example, for the age group [39 - 72], the OR = 1.01 (95% CI: 0.92, 1.13).

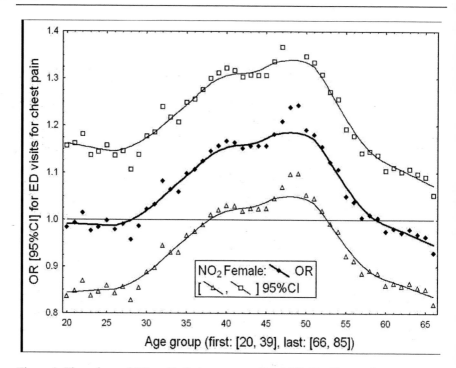

Figure 1. The values of ORs with their corresponding 95% CIs. The results are shown for 47 age groups.

Discussion

In this study, significant short-term effects on daily ED visits for chest pain for females in Toronto were observed as a result of nitrogen dioxide exposure. Ambient air pollution affects patients in different age ranges [6]. This can be the result of different daily behaviour and/or different health status. It should be noted that the overlapping age intervals method identifies the age interval ([39- 72]) for the patients affected by NO_2 exposure. The results suggest that higher air pollution levels (large median values) and acute air pollution events (large Q3) might result in an elevated number of ED visits for chest pain. The results were not statistically significant for the predefined age groups (all, <66 years, 65+ years).

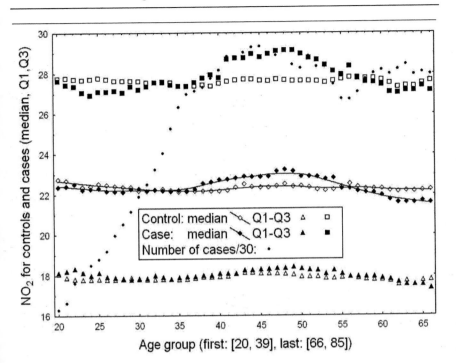

Figure 2. Median, 25th (Q1) and 75[Th] (Q3) percentiles for controls and cases (NO$_2$ in ppb), and the number of cases (divided by 30). The results are shown for 47 age groups.

The recent literature identifies more new health outcomes that are correlated with ambient air pollution exposure [6]. However, a predefined sequence of age intervals, as it was shown, may result in a "leak" in detection of positive and statistically significant results. In our example, no significant results were obtained for the age groups 'all', < age 66, and age 65+.

The limitations of this study are typical of this type of research. They include the adequacy of the applied model and the impact of measurement error in the exposure and outcome variables. As well, ED visits for chest pain may be differently classified. We also have conducted numerous hypothesis tests, thus increasing the risk of false positive results.

The results support the hypothesis that female ED visits for chest pain are correlated with exposure to ambient nitrogen dioxide concentrations. They also indicate a specific age range ([39 – 72]) in which the significant effect was observed. This interval was estimated on the basis of used data, and it is not a universal conclusion. The author suggests designating the term 'continuous age intervals (CAI) methodology', or the CAI method, for the approach presented here to identify age intervals.

Acknowledgments

The author appreciates the efforts of Health Canada in securing these data and for funding data acquisition. The author acknowledges Environment Canada for providing the air pollution data from its National Air Pollution Surveillance network.

References

[1] Szyszkowicz M. Air pollution and ED visits for chest pain. *Am. J. Emerg. Med.* 2009 Feb;27(2):165-168.

[2] Szyszkowicz M., Rowe BH. Air pollution and emergency department visits for chest pain and weakness in Edmonton, Canada. *Int. J. Occup. Med. Environ. Health.* 2010;23:15-19.

[3] Maclure M. The case-crossover design: a method for studying transient effects on the risk of acute events. *Am. J. Epidemiol.* 1991;133:144-153.

[4] Janes H., Sheppard L., Lumley T. Case-crossover analyses of air pollution exposure data. Referent selection strategies and their implications for bias. *Epidemiology* 2005;166:717-726.

[5] World Health Organization. *The International Classification of Diseases, 9th Revision.* Geneva: WHO;1997.

[6] Larrieu S., Lefranc A., Gault G., Chatignoux E., Couvy F., Jouves B., Filleul L.. Are the short-term effects of air pollution restricted to cardiorespiratory diseases? *Am. J. Epidemiol.* 2009;169(10):1201-1208.

Index

D

E

T